FITNESS *over 40*

FITNESS
over 40

A SIX-WEEK EXERCISE PLAN
to Build Endurance, Strength, and Flexibility

Stefanie Lisa

Illustrations by Mat Edwards

**ROCKRIDGE
PRESS**

This book is dedicated to my rock, my knight in shining Under Armour, Larry Waters. Without your constant support and love, none of this would have been possible, and I thank God every day for having you in my life. I love you.

For general information on our other products and services or to obtain technical support, please contact our Customer Care Department within the United States at (866) 744-2665, or outside the United States at (510) 253-0500.

Rockridge Press publishes its books in a variety of electronic and print formats. Some content that appears in print may not be available in electronic books, and vice versa.

TRADEMARKS: Rockridge Press and the Rockridge Press logo are trademarks or registered trademarks of Callisto Media Inc. and/or its affiliates, in the United States and other countries, and may not be used without written permission. All other trademarks are the property of their respective owners. Rockridge Press is not associated with any product or vendor mentioned in this book.

Interior and Cover Designer: Jami Spittler
Art Producer: Hannah Dickerson
Editor: Jesse Aylen

Illustrations © Mat Edwards
Decorative pattern used under license from Shutterstock.com

ISBN: Print 978-1-64876-971-9
eBook 978-1-64876-279-6

R0

CONTENTS

INTRODUCTION

Thank you for choosing this book and making a commitment to better your health and fitness. While everyone has their own individual reasons for starting their fitness journey, this book is designed to meet you where you are now and guide you through a program that you can tailor to your needs.

I'm passionate about helping others become their best selves through fitness and healthy habits. As a Certified Personal Trainer and Life Coach with a certification in Fitness Nutrition as well as 30 years of experience under my weight belt, I'm uniquely qualified to help you harness your motivation and reach your potential. I want to show you how you can improve your life, boost your confidence, and get your groove back by making fitness and health a top priority.

In this book, you will discover practical ways to:

→   Begin a fitness regimen
→   Regain your fitness
→   Maintain your fitness

As you go through this book, you'll find that each exercise comes with tips for adjusting your workouts to your changing needs. When combined, the exercises will enable you to protect and bolster your strength, flexibility, vitality, and freedom.

Most important, always take your own unique needs into account before beginning any fitness regimen. The exercises, nutritional tips, supplement suggestions, and fitness advice in this book are intended for healthy adults to use only after consulting with your primary care doctor. Everyone is different, so remember to take things at your own pace.

Last, your health is the most precious gift you can give, not only to yourself, but to your loved ones as well. Congratulations for committing yourself to better health and deciding to live powerfully for decades to come! I'm excited to be taking this journey with you.

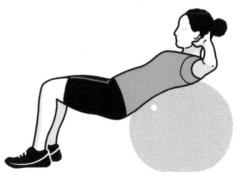

PART 1

A Solid Start

In part 1, we'll learn how four key types of training—endurance, resistance, flexibility, and balance—can benefit our bodies no matter our age. We'll discuss the obstacles in the way of realizing your fitness goals and discover practical strategies to make fitness a priority, whether you're struggling with motivation, working within a budget, or are simply unsure about how to get started. Finally, we'll explore how to eat to fuel our workouts, what supplements and vitamins may help our bodies, and what accessible fitness tools and gear to have on hand.

Let's get started!

1

AGING AND YOUR BODY

This chapter will help you understand how your body changes over time, the value of getting fit, and the importance of maintaining a fitness practice throughout your life. Together, we'll also explore different types of training and why each one is beneficial to building and maintaining your strength, fitness, and vitality.

Fitness after 40

Everyone will start to notice a change in their bodies as they age, whether they're just hitting 40 or crossed that proverbial hill long ago. How those changes manifest will be different for everyone, but most people will notice one or more of the following:

→ Difficulty losing weight
→ Decreased flexibility
→ Joint pain
→ Difficulty lifting heavy objects
→ Decreased muscle tone
→ Weight gain in unexpected areas
→ Becoming more easily winded with less exertion

These slight changes are a normal part of living, but with exercise and a healthy lifestyle, you can minimize—and perhaps even reverse—some of these effects.

When it comes to the importance of exercise and how your body functions, it's often a case of "use it or lose it." In 1966, the University of Texas Southwestern Medical School conducted a study in which five healthy 20-year-old men were confined to bed rest for three weeks. In that short period, these men increased their body fat, lost muscle mass, and exhibited troubling health markers such as higher blood pressure and an increased resting heart rate.

Fortunately, there's a silver lining. When these same young men were put on a two-month workout regimen, they not only *reversed* those effects, but also *improved* all their health markers. The takeaway: You can improve your health and fortify your body against aging with a consistent exercise program whether you're committing to it at home, in the gym, or wherever works best for you. No matter your age, it's never too late to start.

Endurance Training

Endurance training is cardiovascular or aerobic activity that elevates your heart rate and gets you moving on a regular basis. You can increase your endurance through activities like walking, biking, swimming, jogging, and using rowing and elliptical machines.

When committing to endurance training, focus on the concepts of pulse, power, and pace. You want your heart rate (pulse) to be in the target zone for your age, to pack some power behind your movement, and to keep up a steady rhythmic pace.

If you're new to endurance exercise, you might be wondering where to start. Let's imagine you're training for a marathon. Training properly would require shorter running workouts that progressively lead to longer workouts, covering more distance until you are able to run the full marathon without stopping. It would require that you commit to endurance training over time to improve your cardiovascular performance.

Recall those young men from the Dallas study who were able to undo the damage done from three weeks of bed rest. Thirty years later, after going through the "normal" aging process, they reconvened with the researchers and were put on an endurance-training program to improve their health. After completing that program, not only did the men lose body fat and bring their health markers back to normal levels; they also surpassed their earlier fitness levels from their 20s! That's the power of an endurance-training program.

Heart Health

Think of your heart as another muscle that needs to be challenged to get stronger. Though it's always best to check with your doctor first, especially if you've had heart issues in the past, most physicians will recommend some form of endurance training to bolster your heart health. Even the American Heart Association recommends endurance training as one of several types of exercise you should be performing regularly to get and stay healthy. Consider starting slowly and working your way up to 30 minutes a day, five days a week, of moderate aerobic activity.

Stamina

Stamina is how long you can continue to perform an exercise with correct and proper form before exhaustion. The terms *endurance* and *stamina* are often interchanged, but when you think of stamina, think *steady*. Being able to keep up your pace over time is the goal.

Developing stamina takes regular cardiovascular training, but it's something you can build upon. Just as you'd need to start training for that marathon with shorter runs, you'll want to build up your stamina over many workouts.

Try starting with as little as 15 minutes of cardiovascular exercise and adding one to three minutes every time you work out. This type of gentle progression allows your heart and body to get stronger without noticing a huge change in exertion.

Resistance Training

Resistance training (also called weight lifting) involves using a weight such as a barbell, a dumbbell, or even your own body weight to strengthen different muscles. When you lift and lower weights, stress is placed upon the corresponding muscle, which will strengthen that muscle and its surrounding muscle groups over time.

It's in the tearing down of the muscle fibers through weight lifting, and the body's natural and subsequent repair of those tissues, that allows for muscle mass to be built. Muscle mass is "metabolically active" tissue, meaning that it requires calories just to stay alive. Other tissues, like body fat, can thrive without extra calories. This is an important distinction, because the more muscle tissue you have and develop throughout your life, the stronger you and your metabolism will be. With a stronger metabolism, you'll burn more body fat and calories daily because your caloric needs will be higher, resulting in tighter, stronger, and more toned muscles.

Muscle Mass

Your body is composed of lean body mass and body fat. Lean body mass encompasses everything other than body fat: things like bones, muscles, organs, tendons, ligaments, and fluids. As you age, you naturally start to lose a little bit of muscle mass every year, tipping the balance in favor of body fat. Therefore, your weight may remain consistent, but you might feel a bit softer and notice fat storage in new places. The good news is that this can be reversed with resistance training.

When thinking about starting a resistance-training routine, there are some major areas of the body to consider. The main muscle groups are:

→ Chest
→ Shoulders
→ Triceps
→ Back
→ Biceps
→ Legs (quadriceps and hamstrings), glutes, and calves
→ Abdominals

There are many ways to activate these different muscle groups, but some of the most common methods are:

Full-body training: performing one or more exercises for every muscle group during the same workout.

Upper/lower body training: alternating between working muscles in the upper body (chest, shoulders, triceps, back, biceps) on "upper" days and muscles in the lower body, such as legs, glutes (buttocks and hips), calves, and abdominals, on "lower" days.

Push and pull movements: alternating exercises such as push-ups to activate the chest and triceps and pulling movements like pull-ups that use your back and biceps.

Bro split: working out your chest, shoulders, and triceps on one day; back and biceps on another day; and legs, calves, and abs on the third day to round out the muscle groups.

You can split the body parts up however you like (there are many variations on these suggestions we'll explore later). The main point is to work each area equally in relation to the others to prevent injuries and to maintain balance, stability, and symmetry throughout your body.

Bone Health

Resistance training helps strengthen bones and prevent or slow osteoporosis. As we get older, our bones become more porous and brittle. Combined with proper nutrition and a vitamin or supplement regimen, incorporating resistance training into your fitness practice can make a significant beneficial impact on the health of your bones. Resistance training fosters bone growth in much the same way that it increases muscle density. The stress of the muscle tissues pulling on bones stimulates them to bulk up, and stronger bones are healthier bones.

Flexibility Training

If you think about a sapling, you'll likely picture a flexible tree that can withstand wind and rain to grow into a stronger, stable tree. Like saplings, we can fall, twist, turn, and bend when we're young, but our ability to do so changes as we get older; our joints get stiffer, and our muscles, tendons, and ligaments become less pliable. This stiffness may limit our range of motion, increasing the possibility of injury. That's why doing what we can to maintain our flexibility is paramount to our overall health.

Agility

If you want to live a more varied life with fewer aches and pains, being agile is key. *Agility* is defined as possessing dexterity and nimbleness, which is slightly different from flexibility. Being agile means that you can move and change positions quickly. Think of a football player; someone who is agile and can stop at a specific moment, change directions quickly, and jump out of the way, all without losing balance or even slowing down.

The ability to move your body quickly and easily through different planes of movement comes from practicing agility training. Many functional movements incorporate some degree of agility, like stooping to pick something up, avoiding obstacles, catching something if you drop it, and being able to twist and move without injury.

Movement

Moving is just as important, if not more so, as our bodies age, but if you don't *stay* active, it can be difficult to get up and running again. Maintaining movement is vital not only for lifestyle reasons, but also because regular activity increases blood circulation throughout your body. Better circulation means faster healing, a stronger immune system, more energy, and a wider range of mobility, which can result in improved cardiovascular health and a stronger metabolism.

Balance Training

Balance is about being able to control your body, whether in motion or while stationary. Balance is also about ensuring that all your muscles are equally strong, allowing you to feel stable and maintain good posture. Some notable benefits of better balance training include:

→ Improved muscle tone
→ Stronger bones

→ Less dizziness
→ Better posture
→ Enhanced coordination

Avoid Injuries

Good balance gives you the advantage when it comes to avoiding injuries. When balanced, your body is aligned and symmetrical so that you can function equally on both sides. Consider a misaligned vehicle with uneven wear and tear on the tires and body. Any mechanic could tell you that a poorly aligned vehicle will cause myriad degenerative problems. Much like that misaligned car, your body is susceptible to injury when out of balance, making it more likely that you'll overcompensate for weaker areas by taxing the more dominant areas as you move through daily activities and exercise. Over time, this type of overuse can lead to serious injuries.

Prevent Falls

Standing upright and moving freely was probably your normal operating mode when you were younger. But, as you age, your ability to stay balanced might not come as naturally. Avoiding a fall in the first place should be your top priority. When your body maintains a stable stance and position, your chances of falling are significantly reduced, which is essential as you get older, because a fall can result in broken bones, sprains, and other debilitating injuries.

Studies show that for improving balance, it's important to have a regular fitness program that includes strength, flexibility, and mobility training. Fall-prevention programs that include each of those exercise modes show great progress in helping older adults avoid falls and the accompanying fractures, allowing them to live more vibrant, self-reliant lives.

Decade-by-Decade Breakdown

Although exercise should remain a constant throughout your life, your needs and abilities will change over time. Recognizing the types of changes you may be facing will allow you to adapt appropriately within your fitness practices as your life progresses.

40s

In your 40s, you may start to notice a bit of a change across the board. As your body has aged, what worked for you in the past isn't quite as potent in the present. This means you need to work out a little smarter (and maybe even a little harder) to maintain your overall fitness level.

Hormone levels can also be major players in your overall fitness. Your levels of estrogen and/or testosterone may have decreased, and now perhaps it seems as if even glancing at a piece of cake will make you feel 10 pounds heavier. Those fluctuations usually mean that your body is changing the way it metabolizes and stores fat.

To help counteract these changes, stick with regular workouts (or get started again) and incorporate resistance training into your routine several times a week. Practice developing a mind-body connection by focusing on the muscle you are working. Feel and hold each muscle contraction, making every repetition count.

50s

Cardiovascular health becomes a priority in your 50s, and a reliable, regular aerobic program is essential for maintaining heart health. While it's still important to continue strength, flexibility, and balance training, committing to a cardiovascular-boosting endurance routine should be your top priority.

You may also notice that it's taking you a bit longer to recover from exercise. This is a normal occurrence, and most likely due to not pushing yourself hard enough on a regular basis over the years. To overcome longer recovery periods, incorporate flexibility training and stretching exercises into every workout. Otherwise, your body will never be able to progress.

Finally, continue with weight-bearing exercises. Resistance training is vital, especially for women, when it comes to protecting bones and staving off osteoporosis. Walking and running are great ways to improve and maintain bone density, as well.

60s

In your 60s, joint health should be a priority. Activity spurs circulation, which delivers healing nutrients to stressed joints, allowing them to repair and replenish. Lubricated joints are happy joints, so maintain your aerobic and stretching exercises. Aim to include low-impact exercises like swimming, bicycling, walking, using an elliptical machine, or doing yoga or Tai Chi.

Additionally, be mindful to include weight training. As we get older, our bodies experience the loss of muscle mass and related strength (a phenomenon called sarcopenia), which can only be slowed by regularly lifting weights. Aim to do resistance training three or more times a week and use a progressive style of lifting, making your workout a little more challenging every time by adding weight, reducing rest times, or increasing the number of repetitions you do.

70s

Your 70s are a great time to stay active at the proper pace and enjoy exercise with loved ones. Tennis, golfing, walking, and swimming are just a few of the fun things you can do. Continue doing the things you love while recognizing that you may need a little extra recovery time, or you may need to slow it down a notch or two to avoid overexertion or injury.

If you get fatigued too quickly, you may need longer breaks between exercises, especially if it takes you a little bit longer to warm up and cool down than it used to. Use this extra time to focus on your balance and flexibility exercises. Staying limber is the name of the game.

80s

In your 80s, use strength training for muscle preservation and healthy bone density, coupled with balance and flexibility regimens for a well-rounded routine. Continuing your fitness program is a must if your goal is to maintain your independence.

Train at your own pace and be sure to monitor your heart rate in addition to other health factors. Take extra rest time as needed, allow for more recovery between workouts, and move at an easy pace, especially if you're navigating other physical challenges. You have what it takes to prevent muscle loss and stay strong.

90s

Strength training is still a benefit, even in your 90s! At this point, you should be focusing on quality of life by fostering your self-reliance and confidence. Consult with a trainer to help you with exercises, monitor your heart rate as you continue your cardiovascular workouts, and never stop working on improving your balance and flexibility.

One study published in *Clinical Interventions in Aging* showed that people in their 70s, 80s, and 90s can still make a difference in their health in the weight room. The study, which involved nursing home residents, revealed that muscle strength and mobility could be vastly improved with just two sessions of weight training a week. Strength training, especially for the lower body, helps combat age-related muscle loss and reduces the incidence and likelihood of falls.

Overall Brain Health

According to a study published by the American Academy of Neurology (AAN), regular physical exercise significantly contributes to a healthy mind and can even help prevent dementia. In this

20-year study, participants were given a movement tracker to assess their physical activity for 24 hours a day. Those who engaged in regular activity outshone their sedentary counterparts on cognition and memory tests. Moreover, researchers discovered that even a slight increase in physical activity produced up to a 31 percent decrease in the likelihood of developing dementia.

In another study, also published by the AAN, 160 elderly participants with slight cognitive decline were divided into four groups: those who followed a healthy diet, those who only received education about their health, those who followed a three-day-a-week aerobic program, and those who followed both the diet and the exercise programs. The participants who followed both programs for six months had the best cognitive results, while those following the exercise-only regimen came in a close second.

Finally, exercise has been proven to increase the size of the hippocampus, a part of the brain involved in short-term, long-term, and spatial memory. A 2011 National Academy of Sciences study found that aerobic exercise was instrumental in reversing age-related memory loss by more than a year while increasing the size of the hippocampus by 2 percent.

TAKEAWAYS

Our bodies change as we age, and those changes can affect everything we do. From hormone fluctuations to changes in body composition and overall health, having a solid fitness plan in place is key to optimal longevity.

There are a few main areas of focus that you should include in your exercise regimen:

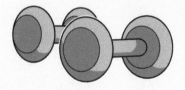

→ Endurance training
→ Resistance training
→ Flexibility training
→ Balance training

It's important to recognize that your needs will change as you move through the decades. A program that worked for you in the past may need to be modified according to your current needs to maintain its effectiveness. Always keep in mind the significant beneficial impact that a fitness lifestyle can have on your physical and brain health.

2

OBSTACLES TO YOUR FITNESS

This chapter will help you explore the roadblocks that may have stopped you from getting fit or derailed your fitness plans. You'll learn what to do if you feel out of shape, can't fit exercise into your schedule, are worried about cost, or simply don't know where to start.

What If I'm Out of Shape?

Everyone begins somewhere, and the sooner you start, the further ahead you'll be before you know it. According to scientists, as little as one week away from exercise can cause a sharp downturn in your level of fitness. But don't worry if it's been longer than that. Scientists also say that as little as 30 minutes of walking, five times a week, can boost your fitness levels in no time. Here are two simple strategies that will get you going again.

Strategy #1: Start Slowly

Just as you wouldn't run a marathon without training, you shouldn't jump into a high-intensity exercise program all at once. Start slowly, maybe by just walking around the block. Adding three short minutes a day, if you walk five days a week, will have you bumping yourself up in 15-minute increments every week.

When you're ready, try adding some resistance training. Aim to lift weights at least twice a week until you get accustomed to the exercises. Stick with moderate repetitions (such as 15 per exercise) and make it heavy enough to feel, but not so heavy that you can't complete all 15 reps. Over the next few months, gauging how you feel, increase the weight and the number of workouts per week.

Strategy #2: Join a Fitness Challenge

Fitness challenges are a fun way to get motivated, learn from others, and boost one another during your respective fitness journeys. To find them, try your local gym, community center, or check out online fitness sites. Supplement companies and dieting websites also hold contests to help you get in better shape. January is the most popular time to join a fitness challenge, followed by spring and summer months, but any time you're ready is the perfect time to start.

You may be intimidated about going to the gym after such a long time away, but taking the first step is the biggest hurdle. Joining up with others who also may have let their fitness slip is a great way to get back into the swing of things. You can negotiate the experience together as a group and share thoughts, feelings, motivations, and ideas along the way.

What If I Don't Have Time?

You make time for what's important to you, and not taking care of you is a way of telling yourself that you're not that important. Make yourself, and your health, a priority.

Getting fit and staying healthy can make you a happier, calmer, and more balanced person overall. When you make the time for your workouts, you'll be more productive and confident, less stressed and depressed, and more energized. Here are two strategies to help you get it done.

Strategy #1: Set Appointments with Yourself

Things that are a priority tend to get done. Your exercise needs to be scheduled, just like any other critical appointment. You wouldn't dream of missing an important meeting or doctor's visit, so you shouldn't miss your workouts, either.

Blocking off the time you need to exercise makes it a real thing. Once you put it on the calendar, it becomes important and everything else fills in the time slots around it. Try making a standing appointment with yourself and the gym, or even with your home workout setup, and see how easy it is to develop the habit of sticking to it. Later, we'll explore how to make either, or both, of these workout habits a constant reality with structured workout plans.

Strategy #2: Do More Efficient Workouts

This is one instance where multitasking is not a bad thing once you have proper exercise form in place. Watching your favorite television shows while walking on the treadmill? Great! Reading a book while pedaling on the recumbent bike? Fantastic. These are just two of many ways to take care of business.

Doing compound movements at the gym can also accomplish a lot in a short amount of time. Compound movements are exercises that require the use of several muscle groups at once to complete the movement. For example, push-ups will use your chest muscles, but also your shoulders, triceps, abdominals, and other muscles in your core.

Another option is to try some circuit training. Circuit training involves doing about 8 to 10 exercises, alternating which muscles you're working at each "station." You'll likely also do some form of cardiovascular exercise between the resistance exercises like step-ups, jump rope, biking, and more. You'll not only work the muscles of your entire body, but if you keep up the pace, you can incorporate cardio at the same time.

If all else fails, give your daily movements an extra boost: park farther away from your office, take the stairs, learn to fidget, and become extremely inefficient with your movements (like getting up repeatedly to take a single piece of paper out of the printer). These small activities can add up to a surprisingly large amount of extra movement throughout the day, taking you even further in your larger fitness goals.

What If I Don't Have the Money?

There are many ways to get in a workout without spending a lot of money. These days, there is a wide variety of options at your fingertips, making it even easier to start a fitness program. Even if your budget is a bit tight, check out these strategies to try out a workout free or at a nominal cost.

Strategy #1: Home Workouts

Now, more than ever before, we have ways of getting in shape without leaving the house and certainly without having to go to the gym.

Go online! Check out YouTube for free programs and tutorials. Or you can find other guided workouts and training series for very little investment. Simply look up "body weight workouts" and you will immediately have many options at your fingertips.

Also, don't forget the great outdoors. You can always walk, run, or bike and throw in some push-ups and crunches for an effective, yet free, workout.

Strategy #2: Group Training

When you have to go it alone, things can get expensive, but when you team up with other people who share your fitness goals, things suddenly become much more affordable (and fun!).

Training with a group is also great if you don't know exactly what to do, need a little boost in motivation, or need some accountability.

If you want to step things up a notch, consider hiring a personal trainer with two, three, or four friends. Splitting the cost among the entire group can make this kind of training affordable, and you can learn a lot while still getting plenty of individualized attention and instruction.

What If I Don't Know What I'm Doing?

You don't have to know what you're doing to get started. In fact, it's almost a certainty that nobody knows what they're doing when they first embark on their fitness journey! It's a learning process, and everyone goes through it. The important thing is simply to start.

Strategy #1: Learn from Watching

Imitation is the sincerest form of flattery, and that holds true in the fitness arena as well. When you're just starting out and everything seems unfamiliar, you may want to start with something easy, like a treadmill or elliptical machine. While using that machine, you can observe how others are using the equipment around you and then try to copy their movements.

Try to emulate the movements of someone who clearly knows what they're doing based on their fitness or experience level. If you're up to it, you can ask them what they're doing and how.

Another great way to learn is by watching videos online. You can type an exercise into any video streaming site (such as YouTube), and a host of selections will explain how to do the exercise. Keep reading for a broad range of exercises and proper techniques in the later chapters.

Strategy #2: Invest in a Trainer

If your budget allows for it, investing in a knowledgeable, experienced trainer is one of the best things you can do to attain your fitness goals. A trainer can help you navigate your way around a gym and teach you which exercises to perform for each muscle group and the proper way to do those exercises.

A little-known secret is that everyone gets intimidated at a new gym. That's where a trainer becomes invaluable. Not only will they take the mystery out of the whole process, but more important, they'll ensure that you learn the proper use of machines and practice correct form when doing your exercises.

What If I'm Not Motivated Enough?

If you're not feeling motivated enough to work out, that's probably due to not having a strong enough "why." Here are a couple of simple strategies to help fire up your motivation.

Strategy #1: Finding Your "Why"

What is a "why"? Well, let's begin by imagining a journey with no destination in mind. How will you know when you get there? How will you know if you're on the right path?

The Japanese concept of *ikigai* can help you find your purpose and your why. Its literal translation is "a reason for being," and it starts with you determining your values, your passions, your personal mission, your strengths, and your weaknesses. Think about these principles to find your "why" for your fitness goals. Do you want to stay healthy so you can play with your grandchildren? Maybe living on your own is important and you want to be self-sufficient for as long as possible.

Whatever your reasons, use them to propel yourself into action whenever your motivation flags.

Strategy #2: Accountability Partners

Saying your goals out loud, especially when you commit to them in front of others, makes them real. When you're held accountable by a friend or loved one, you persevere simply because you don't want to let anyone down. Yes, it would be bad enough to let yourself down, but the possibility of losing face and disappointing others is extra motivation to keep working toward your goals until you accomplish them.

Remember, where there's a will (and a why!), there's a way.

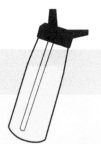

TAKEAWAYS

In this chapter, you learned:

→ What to do if you're out of shape

→ How to make time for exercise by making it a priority

→ How to work out for low or no cost

→ How to figure out what to do through emulation and research

→ How to get motivated to work out by focusing on your "whys"

3

FOUNDATION FOR SUCCESS

In this chapter, we will delve into the foods that will fuel your workouts so you can achieve your goals and maintain optimal health. Together, we'll dig into how different kinds of nutrients can help support your fitness journey.

We'll also discuss how to assess your fitness level as well as what kinds of equipment might be helpful to have on hand and how to work out effectively within your home or a gym. Finally, we'll explore the concepts of rest and recovery, specifically why it's important to give your body some downtime to heal.

Nutrition

When you embark on the six-week exercise plan, you'll want to ensure you're giving your body the building blocks it needs to build lean muscle tissue. Foods are divided up into macronutrient groups: protein, carbohydrates, and fats. How much of each nutrient you need will vary based on your fitness and health goals, sex, age, height, weight, and activity levels.

You can find macronutrient and calorie calculators online at various dieting and fitness websites (check out the Resources section on page 203 for suggestions). Use these to determine your level of maintenance calories (how many calories you need per day just to maintain your current weight). From there, you can also determine how many calories to cut if you want to lose weight, how to decide your macronutrient breakdown, and much more.

Protein Intake

Protein intake is critical when it comes to building a strong body since it forms the building blocks of muscle tissue and helps your body repair and replenish itself. Protein is found in meat, dairy, seafood, beans, lentils, nuts and nut butters, tofu, tempeh, quinoa, wild rice, oatmeal, and vegetables such as spinach, broccoli, and sprouts.

The Food and Nutrition Board of the National Academy of Sciences recommends approximately 0.36 gram of protein per pound of body weight (protein has four calories per gram). However, you can (and should) safely consume additional protein if you are training with weights, participating in a weight-loss program, or both. Again, you can adjust those amounts based on your doctor's recommendations, your activity levels, and your fitness goals.

Carbohydrate Intake

Carbohydrate intake may vary, but a good rule of thumb is to get between 45 and 65 percent of your diet from this category. Carbs, like protein, also have four calories per gram. Carbohydrates are found in potatoes, sweet potatoes, oatmeal, rice, bread, fruits, dairy, nuts, seeds, and legumes.

Carbohydrates can be broken down into distinct categories: sugars, starches, and fiber. Fruits and dairy products have a lot of sugars (fructose, sucrose, and lactose), and are useful as energizing pre-workout meals. Vegetables, beans, and grains have starch and fiber, and are great for helping you replenish post-workout. Depending on your individual fitness and health goals, you may consider focusing on fiber-rich, whole-grain foods and low-sugar and low-fat carb choices.

Fat Intake

At nine calories per gram, you'll want to keep a close eye on your fat intake and choose healthy fats like monounsaturated and polyunsaturated fats found in avocados, olives and olive oils, nuts and nut butters, seeds, and fatty fish such as salmon, mackerel, sardines, and trout.

Steer clear of artificial trans fats found in prepackaged snack foods, fried foods, cakes, cookies, pastries, and foods containing hydrogenated vegetable oil. Consider limiting your consumption of saturated fats to those in meats, full-fat dairy products, and oils. Try to keep your fat intake to between 20 and 35 percent of your total calories.

Breakfast

For a healthy boost of energy, consider breakfasts that contain protein, healthy carbohydrates, and a small amount of fat. Some options include:

→ Oatmeal and blueberries with almond butter
→ Whole wheat toast with half a sliced avocado
→ Greek yogurt with strawberries and almond slivers
→ Half a grapefruit and Ezekiel bread with peanut butter

→ Whole-grain cereal with sliced banana and almond milk
→ Scrambled egg whites, one whole egg, reduced-fat cheese, Ezekiel bread

Lunch

Lunch should be a balanced meal of moderate protein, moderate carbohydrates, and medium fats. Consider choices like:

→ Boneless, skinless grilled chicken breast with a baked sweet potato and green beans
→ Whole wheat tortilla wrap with flaked tuna, lettuce, and light dressing
→ Pan-seared chicken breast in a whole wheat tortilla with grilled peppers and onions
→ Baked tofu with mixed vegetables
→ Shredded baked chicken over quinoa with a side salad and low-sugar barbecue sauce
→ Grilled sirloin steak with broccoli and a baked potato

Dinner

Keep your last meal of the day low-fat, low-carb, and high-protein. Think about options such as:

→ Baked boneless, skinless chicken breast with broccoli
→ Grilled salmon with wild rice and a side salad
→ Grilled lean pork with red and green peppers over rice
→ Pan-seared tofu with roasted carrots and spinach
→ Grilled shrimp with quinoa and a diced cucumber salad
→ A large baked red pepper stuffed with red beans and jasmine rice

Pre-Workout

Before a workout, you'll want to eat lightly, getting in protein and carbohydrates while skimping on fats. The carbs will provide energy quickly, while the protein will give your muscles the nutrients to repair themselves after exercise. Consider snacking on these before your next workout:

→ Nonfat Greek yogurt with blueberries
→ A protein shake with half an apple
→ Cottage cheese with berries
→ A banana and a glass of almond milk
→ An apple with low-fat string cheese
→ A fruit smoothie with a scoop of protein powder or nut butter

Post-Workout

After your workout, ideally, you'll have some protein, starchy carbs, and fewer fats. The starchy carbs will keep you full and satisfied while allowing your body to replenish the lost glycogen in your bloodstream. Satisfy yourself with:

→ Oatmeal mixed with protein powder and one tablespoon of peanut butter
→ Handful of almonds, an apple, and one scoop of whey protein blended with one cup of almond milk
→ Diced grilled chicken and a baked sweet potato
→ Half a cup of beans and half a cup of rice with mixed vegetables
→ Greek yogurt with one scoop of protein powder and one tablespoon of almond butter
→ Cottage cheese and mixed berries with whole wheat toast and almond butter

Hydration

It's vital that you drink plenty of fresh water every day. While plain water is best, you can also hydrate with seltzer; water-filled foods like celery, watermelon, and cucumber; and other liquids such as sports drinks. If you're not a fan of unflavored water, add cucumbers, oranges, berries, lemons, or limes. Aim to consume at least eight 8-ounce glasses of water every day—and much more if you're in a warmer climate, you're exercising, or you sweat frequently.

Supplements

Supplements are designed to fill in nutritional gaps as you continue your workout program.

Multivitamins and minerals: These provide simple insurance against nutrient deficiencies. You want to give yourself all the tools you need to stay healthy and keep your immune system strong.

Fish oil: Fish oil, containing omega-3 fatty acids that boost heart health, is an anti-inflammatory supplement that can keep your brain healthy and eyesight sharp. Scientists say fish oil may even protect and stimulate the growth of new muscle tissue.

Vitamin C: Vitamin C helps to keep your immune system strong, protects against heart disease, and keeps your eyes healthy and your skin supple.

Vitamin D: Vitamin D helps keep your bones strong, strengthens your immune system, stabilizes your blood sugar levels, and supports your lungs and heart. Take it with vitamin C and calcium, as it helps with the absorption of those nutrients.

Probiotics: Probiotics ensure that your intestinal flora, the good bacteria in your gut, have a chance to thrive. Healthy gut bacteria can help manage irritable bowel syndrome, ulcerative colitis, and Crohn's disease, as well as bladder and yeast infections.

B vitamins: These vitamins keep your mood swings in check while helping your brain stay sharp. B vitamins also aid in the metabolism of food as it is processed into energy. With a more efficient digestive system, you can manage your weight more easily, get the most out of your dietary choices, and keep your energy levels high.

Fitness Test

Taking a basic fitness test before beginning your fitness program establishes a baseline of where you are starting and ensures that you are healthy and strong enough to begin the protocol.

Ask yourself these questions, answering *Yes* or *No* to each:

1. Do I have a heart condition, high blood pressure, or diabetes? (If so, you should find out if you have certain limitations.)

2. Do I have injuries that could become worse with the use of an exercise program? (If so, consider working with a physical therapist before starting a new regimen.)

3. Do I experience dizziness or loss of balance that could prohibit me from performing any of the exercises in this book?

4. Is my heart rate higher than the average? (Your resting heart rate should be somewhere between 60 and 100 beats per minute. Anything higher could be caused by stress, dehydration, certain medications, or a medical issue.)

5. Have I been prescribed medications or been at risk at any point for high blood pressure?

6. Do I need to clean up my diet?

7. Do I need to focus on my sleep hygiene?

8. Have I exercised in the past and do I know the basics? (If not, it's okay! Everyone starts somewhere.)

9. Can I hold a basic plank (page 84), do a basic squat (page 73), touch my toes, and perform a push-up (page 46)?

10. Can I walk at a moderate pace for 20 minutes?

Results Explained

If you answered Yes to the first five questions and/or No to questions 8, 9, and 10, begin your fitness journey slowly, perhaps with permission from your doctor or with a personal trainer by your side. Especially if you're new to the fitness scene, learning the basics in person from a professional can be key.

Although you may be eager to get started on your fitness journey—and you should be!—setting yourself up for success will pay off in the future. Learning how to improve your health across the board is valuable information that you will use for years to come.

Even if you scored well on the fitness test, it's a good idea to discuss any fitness plans with your doctor. Being healthy isn't a one-size-fits-all process and you may need to accommodate for things like injuries, limitations, medications, and so forth. Finally, don't be discouraged if you're not ready to start today. Getting healthy takes preparation, but it'll all be worth it.

Gear and Equipment List

Having the right tools is essential for success in any endeavor. You wouldn't set out on a camping trip without food, water, shelter, or proper shoes and clothing, so you shouldn't embark on your fitness journey without the proper gear!

Gear List

Having a few inexpensive basics on hand before you start will be immensely helpful.

Clothing: Make sure you're comfortable in your clothes. Dressing in practical clothing that is nonrestrictive, breathable, and wicks away sweat can help keep you comfortable and focused on your exercise program. Consider dressing in layers so you can remove them as needed. If you enjoy wearing loose clothing to the gym, ensure you're not wearing pants that could potentially get trapped in the wheel of a bicycle or snagged on a piece of equipment. Often, people will wear stretchy leggings or shorts that allow for greater movement, or tank tops so that they can observe their upper-body muscles working, helping to solidify that mind-body connection.

Footwear: Having the appropriate footwear depends on the type of activity you're performing. If you're running or jogging regularly, invest in a stable, cushioned running shoe. If you're lifting weights, there are specific flat-soled stable shoes, as well as shoes dedicated for walking, and special shoes just for cycling. Regardless of the activity you choose, it's important to have the shoes you need.

Make sure to also get the right fit! Certain shoes come with extra cushioning or stability to help prevent injuries, which won't work properly if the shoe is too tight or too loose. Ask a salesperson at your local specialty shoe store to help you ensure you have the proper fit.

Weight lifting and other gym accessories: Consider getting a pair of weight lifting gloves to help you grip the equipment. Not only can gloves help strengthen your grip, but they can minimize calluses, and even support your wrists if you opt for gloves with wrist wraps.

Invest in a sturdy gym bag to hold your gym clothes, footwear, water bottle, notebook, and anything else you might need. Bringing your own towels to dry off with or to place on the equipment is also a good idea, as well as a padlock for your locker and flip-flops if you plan to shower.

Music: Lastly, consider getting a pair of headphones or earbuds. There's nothing more motivating than ramping up the energy of your workout with fun music of your choice.

Equipment List

Dumbbells and weights: A well-stocked gym will have a full rack of dumbbells in all the weight increments from light (five pounds or lighter) up to very heavy (at least 100 pounds, if not more).

If you're interested in weight training at home, consider purchasing a small variety of dumbbells, from very light (3 to 5 pounds) up to moderately heavy (20 to 30 pounds), depending on your budget, strength, and goals.

Universal systems: Gyms will often have what's called a "universal" tree or system, which will be equipped with bars for pull-ups and pull-downs, as well as a cable system. If you have the space in your home and want to purchase one of these combo systems, go for it, but it isn't necessary. Many of this book's exercises can be done at home without much equipment at all.

Resistance bands: These stretchy bands can help you get a great workout at home or in the gym without machines or dumbbells. Used to provide resistance for your muscles, they can help you stretch and become stronger and more flexible.

Stability ball: This ball gives you an unstable surface that can help you work your core even as you work other body parts. Stability balls promote stretching and flexibility, help with balance exercises and can even function as a chair or bench for certain moves.

Extras: Don't forget how handy a yoga mat can be! Its padded nonslip surface provides exactly what you need for stretching and floor movements. Also consider getting a jump rope to use for the warm-up portions of your cardio training or for high-intensity interval work.

To improvise in a pinch, use cans and water jugs in place of dumbbells, a staircase, or the outdoors instead of equipment, and your own body weight.

Rest and Recovery

To achieve your goals without injuring or overworking yourself, your body needs both short- and long-term recovery periods, as well as active rest.

Rest

Short-term recovery is the rest in between sets of exercises and your cool-down period. Just as you do a 5- to 10-minute warm-up before your sets, you should also do a 5- to 10-minute cool-down, letting your heart rate and breathing slow, allowing your body to gently transition into rest mode. Cool-downs can include walking, stretching, balance, flexibility moves, and even yoga.

Long-term recovery refers to the days in between working the muscle group or groups in your body. This rest period is also the time when your muscles grow, as opposed to when you are exercising and tearing the fibers down.

Active recovery may sound counterintuitive, but it simply means engaging in other activities throughout your day. For example, you might play a game of basketball, go golfing, or hike with friends on a day that you're not working out.

Sleep

Set your bedroom up for optimal sleep by keeping it as dark, quiet, and cool as possible. Ideal sleeping temperatures will vary based on your preferences, but somewhere between 60 and 67 degrees is a good start. If you have trouble sleeping, adding a magnesium supplement to your diet can help, because it calms your central nervous system.

How to Evaluate

Rest: How do you know if you're getting the right amount of rest? If you are lethargic during the day, it's probably a sign that you may need to get some additional rest. Try having a bedtime ceremony to mentally prepare your mind and to help your body wind down toward the end of the day.

Soreness: An indication of possible overtraining is muscle soreness. It's normal for your muscles to be sore the day after you work them and even 48 hours later. However, if soreness persists for longer than three days after your workout, you may need a little extra time to recover.

Motivation: If you find yourself losing your desire to exercise or just going through the motions, you may need an extra day off to renew that internal fire. Revisit some of your goals and "whys," recharging your internal passion for health and fitness.

Age: As you get older, you may find that you're not recovering as quickly as you once did, which is completely normal. A good rule of thumb to follow is if the muscles you worked are still sore, give them another day and then revisit the possibility of training.

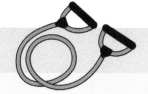

TAKEAWAYS

In this chapter, we discussed:

→ Nutrition and its importance in your general health and overall fitness
→ Discussing fitness plans with your physician
→ The gear and equipment you'll need before you get started
→ The importance of rest and recovery

Your Fitness Routine

In part 2, you'll build on what you learned in part 1 about making fitness a key piece of your lifestyle.

Within the next pages, you'll learn about the different types of training: endurance, resistance, flexibility, and balance. You'll also learn why each type is important for a solid fitness program. You'll be introduced to different exercises that work each muscle group, and they can all be done in your home or at the gym. Finally, you will find a six-week workout program you can customize to your unique needs.

4

ENDURANCE TRAINING

In this chapter, we'll discuss endurance training, including a vast array of exercise options, techniques, and modifications you can explore. You'll discover why it's so important to engage in a full-body program and learn about the vast benefits that endurance training is specifically suited to provide.

Because we'll be reviewing the finer points of specific exercises and discussing proper form, you'll want to mark this section for easy reference, as you will return often to ensure your form is on point and that you're getting the most out of the suggested exercises.

Why Endurance Training?

Endurance training is one-fourth of a well-rounded workout program, which also includes resistance training, flexibility training, and balance work. Endurance training is a form of cardio-vascular exercise, also known as "aerobics" or "cardio." This type of exercise is designed to get your heart rate up and your blood circulating throughout your body.

To ensure you get the most out of your endurance-training sessions, you'll want to get your heart rate between 50 and 85 percent of your maximum heart rate. To get an approximate determination of what that is, subtract your age from 220 then multiply it by .50 and .85, respectively; your maximum heart rate should fall somewhere between those two numbers.

How Much Do I Need?

According to the American Heart Association, healthy adults should be achieving a minimum of 150 minutes of moderate aerobic activity a week, which breaks down to about 30 minutes five days a week or 22 minutes every day. If you're industrious, you can aim for 75 minutes of very intense interval training per week.

But if you're just embarking on your fitness journey and you're not ready to do a dedicated 30-minute session of exercise, start by aiming to move around more than you have been. If you can spend a total of one hour a day, five days a week, just moving about and being active, you'll be doing yourself a huge favor when it comes to raising your fitness level.

Making Progress

When beginning any new program, being at the starting line can be daunting. It takes time, patience, and perseverance to move forward and make gains in any endeavor.

Start slowly by doing a few five-minute sessions throughout the day or by adding a few minutes to your endurance workout every time you do it. Remember, every step you take is a step closer to a healthier, fitter version of you.

HEALTH CONCERNS

If you're recovering from an illness or dealing with health concerns such as a stroke or a cardiac event, you don't need to rule out this type of training. In fact, it will likely be beneficial in helping you avoid future issues, but you should proceed only when your physician deems it appropriate.

If you are part of a supervised rehabilitation program, you may be encouraged to participate in endurance-training types of exercises. Typically, you'll start very slowly, possibly adding only steps a day, until you work your way up to more vigorous exercise.

Endurance Exercises

Endurance training can be mild, moderate, or vigorous depending on how fast you move, the level of resistance involved, and the length of time you work out. There are several ways you can do endurance training and several ways to determine how hard you're working. You can measure your heart rate and plug it into a target heart rate calculator (see Resources on page 203). However, the easiest way to tell if you're working hard enough is to check your breathing. If you're slightly out of breath but can still hold a conversation, you're in the perfect zone for endurance exercise.

Walking

Walking is one of the most basic movements, and it's a wonderful way to get started on a solid endurance-training program. But don't let the innocence of a simple walk fool you. Walking can be as challenging as you make it by changing your pace and the terrain.

Walking is gentler on the body, joints, tendons, and ligaments than running, making it a great form of low-impact exercise. It's an ideal way to recover if you've been battling injuries and it's something you can start slowly, building your way up to longer, more rigorous walks.

Walking

Muscle Groups: Legs (quadriceps, hamstrings, inner and outer thighs, calves) hips and glutes, arms and core (if you pump your arms, you'll also engage your upper body and core)

1. Begin by walking at a comfortable, easy pace to adjust your body to the movement. Once you are adjusted and ready to pick up the pace, start by speeding up your walk until you're walking about 3.5 to 4.0 miles per hour.

2. From there, you can bump up your speed to a "speed walking" or "power walking" level, which is somewhere between 4.5 and 5.5 miles per hour.

Safety Pointers: If you're walking outdoors, practice safe walking by staying in well-lit areas, wearing reflective clothing, walking with others, being mindful of traffic, and wearing sunscreen and the appropriate clothing for the weather. If walking regularly, consider investing in a good pair of walking shoes.

Jogging and Running

Jogging and running are both tremendous when it comes to boosting your endurance.

There are many different types of jogging and running doable both indoors and outdoors. If you want a treadmill experience comparable to running outdoors, set the treadmill at a 1 percent incline to simulate the ground's rougher terrain. If you prefer the outdoors, try running on a track or a trail to ramp up the intensity of your workout.

Jogging and Running

Muscle Groups: Legs (quadriceps, hamstrings, inner and outer thighs, calves), hips and glutes, arms and core

1. Start with a sufficient warm-up. Walk for at least five minutes before setting out, because running can put significant force on your bones, tendons, and ligaments.

2. Your posture should be upright and your arms should swing in a natural, relaxed manner close to your sides. Place one foot in front of the other as you propel yourself off your back foot. You want your foot to land approximately under your body's center as you run.

3. Try to land mid-foot as you run (some people land on their toes, putting undue pressure on the calves, or their heels, which may indicate too long a stride).

4. Start off slow and work your way up to longer and longer sessions. Stretch thoroughly after every run! (Check out page 89 for stretching suggestions.)

Safety Pointers: Having the right kind of shoes is even more important when jogging or running. Consider asking a specialty shoe store salesperson to help you choose the best type of running shoe.

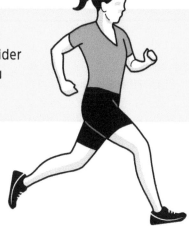

Swimming

Swimming is another fantastic way to get in an endurance workout.

If you're just starting out, consider taking some lessons at a gym, community center, or fitness center if your budget allows it. This is the safest way to build up your skills and perfect your strokes.

Swimming

Muscle Groups: Full body (arms, legs, back, chest, and core)

1. Start by getting comfortable in the shallow end of the pool. Allow your entire body to get wet. Blow bubbles underwater and then stand up and breathe. Repeat this as you move into deeper and deeper water to help build confidence.

2. Move on to floating. Hold your breath, lean backward so your feet come up off the ground of the pool, and allow yourself to float. Next, try the same exercise facedown.

3. After you've mastered this, try using a kickboard. Practice your leg movements by holding onto the board while you scissor kick underwater to move forward.

4. Once you're comfortable with the basics, start swimming for exercise, also known as "doing laps" using strokes like the freestyle (or crawl), breaststroke, backstroke, sidestroke, and butterfly. Pick one or more that you enjoy and try to make it the full length of the pool without stopping.

5. Each session, aim for longer swims without rest. As you get stronger, you'll be able to go farther without stopping.

Safety Pointers: Swim with another adult or a lifeguard on duty. Avoid swimming after a large meal, as cramping may occur, after drinking alcohol, or if taking medications that may impair your judgment and motor skills.

Outdoor Biking and Indoor Cycling

This is a versatile form of endurance exercise that can be done indoors or outside, with others or solo. You can ride a mountain bike or road bike outside, cycle at home on an indoor trainer, or take an indoor cycling class.

If you're new, you may want to start with a cycling class where an instructor will guide you through a workout that includes various intensities and speeds in a group format with motivating music.

Aim for about 30 minutes of pedaling to start, working up to an hour-long class or bike ride. Always start with a 5- to 10-minute warm-up. Pedal easily until your heart rate increases and your muscles loosen, and be sure to stretch after every ride.

Outdoor Biking and Indoor Cycling

Muscle Groups: Legs (quadriceps, hamstrings, calves), hips and glutes, core, back, and arms (for stabilization)

1. Adjust the height of your seat so that when your leg is extended with your foot on the pedal, your knee has a slight bend to it.

2. The handlebars should be easy to reach. If you're bending uncomfortably at the waist or feel as though you're straining to reach the handlebars, move your seat forward.

3. If applicable, test out the brakes and make sure you know how to use them.

4. If your bicycle has gears, start on a low setting and practice switching between gears as you pedal.

Safety Pointers: Wear clothing that will not get trapped in the spinning wheel as you ride. If you're riding outdoors, always be aware of your surroundings. Ride with traffic (not against it) and watch for vehicles.

Elliptical Machines

Elliptical machines are easy on the joints and fun to use. The smooth, impact-free range of motion allows you to always keep your feet on the pedals, which is comfortable for those suffering from injuries or rehabilitating from surgery.

Although the gentle movement may seem easy, you can make your workout more challenging by adjusting the intensity (how fast the pedals are moving), incline (how steep the pedals are), or resistance (how difficult it is to push down the pedal). Most machines are equipped with automatic interval programming, or you can adjust the settings manually to boost your workout difficulty and intensity.

Elliptical Machines

Muscle Groups: Legs (quadriceps, hamstrings, inner and outer thighs, calves), hips and glutes, upper body (some machines will have moving handles that will work your upper body as well)

1. Step up onto the machine and choose your numbered level. Often, there will be a "Quick Start" button you can use.

2. Start with a gentle 5-minute warm-up to loosen your muscles and get your circulation going before picking up the intensity of your workout.

3. Once you are acclimated to the machine, make your workout more challenging by adjusting the intensity, incline, or resistance level.

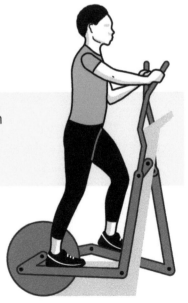

Safety Pointers: Wear clothing that won't get caught in the gears on the machine. Always keep your hands loosely on the handles to maintain your balance.

Rowing

Rowing is an endurance exercise that will raise your heart rate and keep it there. Although it's an excellent cardiovascular workout choice, it can also be an intensive workout and may not be the best starter choice for beginners.

When using a rowing machine, it may take you a while before you can add any resistance at all to your workout. It will take time to build up your stamina on the rower, but that's the name of the game with endurance training!

Rowing

Muscle Groups: Legs, glutes, back, arms, shoulders, and core

1. Rowing is broken into four basic movements: the catch, the drive, the finish, and the recovery.

2. During the catch, your legs should be completely bent as you stretch out your arms and grasp the handle.

3. The drive should be mostly powered by your legs as you push backward and the seat slides with you.

4. The finish lets you use your arms, back, and core to finishing propelling yourself backward.

5. On the recovery, allow your muscles to relax for a moment as you slide the seat forward again to repeat the sequence.

Safety Pointers: Remember to warm up and cool down properly, as a rowing workout is very intense. Take it easy until you get the movements down, as proper form is important.

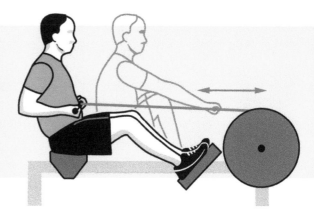

Stair Climbers and Steppers

Stair climbers and steppers are similar to elliptical machines, but somewhat more difficult to master until you get the hang of them. A stair climber has pedals that you "climb" as if standing while pedaling a bike; a stepper (otherwise known as a stepmill) has steps that move much like an escalator as you walk up.

Stair Climbers and Steppers

Muscle Groups: Legs (quadriceps, hamstrings, inner and outer thighs, calves) hips and glutes

1. Step up onto the machine and place each hand comfortably onto the handles.

2. Start with an easy warm-up for about five minutes. Get accustomed to the stepping movement while maintaining a straight, upright posture and resting your hands lightly on the handles. If you find that you're gripping the handles tightly or using them as leverage to pull yourself up, lower your resistance or incline level.

3. When you feel comfortable, increase the speed slowly in short increments until you're out of breath but still able to hold a conversation.

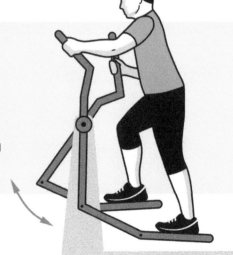

Safety Pointers: If you're a beginner or haven't used a stepper often, avoid TV, books, or visual forms of entertainment until you've familiarized yourself with the equipment and are able to perform the exercise with ease. Be careful when increasing your speed to avoid falling or sustaining a serious injury.

Group Classes

Group classes are an exhilarating way to enhance your aerobic capacity and cardiovascular endurance. Most routines are low-impact and involve stepping up and down on an elevated platform as you follow the instructor's lead, moving your body to the music with dance-like movements that target both legs and arms. You can also enjoy more rigorous boot camp–style classes and martial arts classes such as kickboxing.

Group Classes

Muscle Groups: Full body, depending on the class

1. Always be early! Many classes incorporate some equipment, so you'll want extra time to choose the right equipment and pick a spot where you can clearly see the instructor.

2. Look to your instructor for assistance if you're having trouble or are uncertain of how to perform a specific movement. Your instructor will also be able to help you modify certain exercises to suit your fitness level or accommodate an injury. Always notify the instructor before the class begins if you have any such issues.

3. Don't be afraid to slow down, take breaks, or do a modified version of any exercise. Although you should listen to your instructor, listening to your body first is more important.

4. If the class seems too challenging, don't get discouraged. It usually takes three sessions of a class to get accustomed. If after three classes you're still frustrated, feel free to move on to something else.

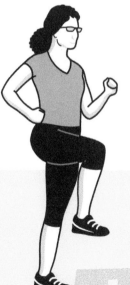

Safety Pointers: Make sure there's enough space between you and your classmates to execute the movements safely. Ensure your water bottle is full before class starts—while there will be breaks between exercises, they're often brief, and staying hydrated is crucial.

5

RESISTANCE TRAINING

It's common to lose muscle mass each year as your body changes. But by incorporating a few strategic resistance-based weight lifting workouts per week into your routine, you can be well on your way to maintaining muscle mass, keeping your metabolism strong, and toning your body.

In this chapter, you'll learn how to maximize your resistance training and which exercises will work best for your fitness needs. You'll also learn all the tips and tricks necessary for maintaining proper form in each exercise.

Why Resistance Training?

Lifting weights and dumbbells or using resistance bands and your own body weight are all forms of resistance training that you'll want to continue throughout your life. Keeping your muscle mass intact and adding new muscle will help you maintain your health, your strength, and your autonomy no matter your age.

How Much Do I Need?

How much weight training you need depends on your fitness level and the types of workouts in which you engage. For a full-body workout, you'll only need two, possibly three, workouts per week. But if you're doing an upper/lower body split, you may need to work out four or even five days a week to exercise all your muscles equally. Regardless of how you choose to structure your workouts, remember to let your muscles rest between sessions so that they can heal and build.

If you're new to weight lifting, you'll probably want to start with two days a week of full-body resistance training. Once your body gets acclimated, you can start adding in extra repetitions or sets, splitting up body parts, and working out with weights more than twice a week. The important thing is to listen to your body and allow yourself to learn the ropes before moving on.

If this sounds like a lot, don't panic! These workouts are designed to be customizable, so you can adjust them until they work for you and your schedule.

Making Progress

Progressive training is something that you can use to get stronger over time. If you think about it, continuing to lift the same amounts, with the same exercises, in the same way year after year will start to yield diminishing results at some point. To keep that plateau from occurring, you can make each consecutive workout a little bit more difficult in some way. Once you've established a comfortable routine, try incorporating some of the following strategies:

→ Increase your weight by half a pound to a few pounds
→ Do a few more repetitions
→ Change your tempo by lifting more slowly
→ Reduce your rest time between sets
→ Work a specific body part more often
→ Try doing high-repetition sets with a lighter weight, such as a set of 50 reps with a five-pound dumbbell

Weights vs. Body Weight

Perk up your exercise program by using weights, as well as your own body weight, in each of your workouts, and note that each has its unique benefits:

Advantages of Training with Weights

→ Greater muscle size over time
→ Increased strength
→ Ability to target specific muscle groups
→ Helps strengthen bones

Advantages of Body-Weight Training

→ Great for beginners who are just learning the ropes
→ Wonderful for at-home workouts with no equipment needed
→ Easy on the joints
→ Helps you learn proper form before progressing to training with weights

Many of the benefits of each type of training overlap each other, so incorporating each kind of training into your workout is your best comprehensive bet.

HEALTH CONCERNS

Working out with proper form is key to preventing injuries. You can start your program even if you have some physical limitations or health issues; you just need to be more strategic with your approach.

If you're new to resistance training, consider hiring a personal trainer or working out with a knowledgeable friend who can show you the ropes. There are also many tutorial videos online if you need to learn how to do certain movements but don't have gym-savvy friends or access to a personal trainer.

Perfecting the proper form early on helps you set the foundation for safe progress. You want to ensure you know how to execute the movements properly so that you can build muscle and lift more weight without getting injured. Doing the movements incorrectly could result in a strain, sprain, or tear. Taking a few minutes at the start to ensure you are practicing good form will go a long way toward keeping you healthy.

Resistance-Training Exercises

The following exercises can be done at home or at the gym. Home workouts will include exercises that use your body weight, as well as basic equipment such as a stability ball, light dumbbells, and resistance bands. Gym workouts will be more varied, because you'll have access to a greater variety of equipment, but home workouts can be equally satisfying and effective.

Chest

Comprising the upper front portion of your torso, your chest muscles are activated through a pushing motion, which is the primary movement in exercises like push-ups, presses, and flies. These exercises will work your chest muscles, as well as some of the smaller surrounding muscle groups like the shoulders and triceps.

REGULAR PUSH-UPS – Body-Weight Exercise (Home or Gym)

Muscle Groups: Chest, shoulders, triceps

1. Begin on your hands and knees with your arms about shoulder width apart and your palms flat on the ground. Your head, back, and hips should form a straight line to your knees. Don't allow your back to hunch over or cave in and keep your hips in line with the rest of your body as you do the movement.

2. Once on your hands and knees, move your legs until they are straight behind you and get up on your toes. Tighten your core and keep your body in a straight line. Ensure that your hips are aligned with your back and legs.

3. Bend your elbows and lower your chest toward the ground until your arms are bent at approximately a 90-degree angle.

4. Using your chest and arms, push back up to starting position by straightening your elbows. You don't need to lock them out at the top of the movement; you can keep a slight bend in your arms. This completes 1 repetition.

5. To make the exercise a little more difficult (and target your triceps), try keeping your elbows closer to your sides throughout the movement.

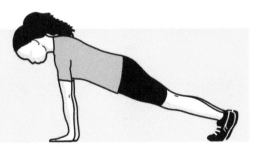

Safety Pointers: Keep your butt down and in line with your body as you complete the movement. Your core should be tight and your back and legs straight.

DUMBBELL CHEST PRESS – Weight Lifting Exercise (Home or Gym)

Muscle Groups: Chest, shoulders, triceps

1. Begin by lying on your back on the floor (if you're at home) or on a bench (if you're at a gym).

2. Select a dumbbell that is light enough that you can do 12 to 15 repetitions, but heavy enough so that the last 5 reps are difficult. You may want to start with a 5- or 10-pound dumbbell and go from there.

3. Grasp a dumbbell in each hand and place your hands, palms facing forward, next to your ears by bending at the elbows. You should feel a nice stretch through your chest area.

4. Push upward by straightening your arms and squeezing your chest muscles, raising the dumbbells up into the air.

5. Once your arms are straight, gently and slowly lower the weight back to starting position. This completes 1 repetition.

Safety Pointer: Never lock out your elbows, and always keep a small bend in them to protect your joints.

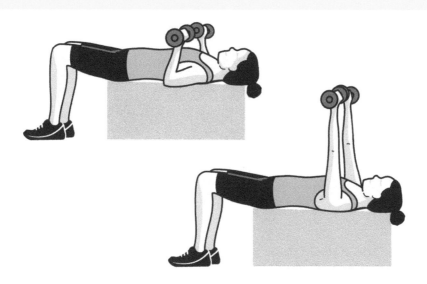

LYING BANDED CHEST PRESS – Band Exercise (Home or Gym)

Muscle Groups: Chest, shoulders, triceps

1. Start by lying on your back with the band on the floor underneath your shoulder blades.

2. Grasp the ends of the band in each hand and bend your arms so your elbows are out to the sides of your body near your ears.

3. Push upward, straightening your arms as you pull the ends of the bands up.

4. Squeeze your chest muscles as you do this motion, keeping your back flat on the ground.

5. Gently lower your elbows back to the ground. This completes 1 repetition.

6. If you need to make the exercise a little more difficult, wrap the band around your hands a few times or simply grab the band farther from the end so that it takes more effort to pull it upward.

Safety Pointer: Make sure you keep the right amount of tension on the band. If it's too loose, you'll get nothing out of the exercise, but if you find yourself straining then it's too tight.

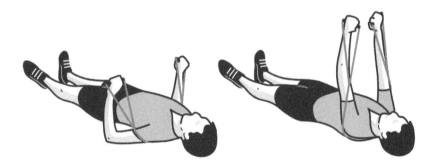

DUMBBELL OR BANDED FLIES – Weight Lifting Exercise (Home or Gym)

Muscle Groups: Chest, shoulders

1. Start by lying on the floor or on a bench if you're at the gym. Place your feet on the ground with your knees bent.

2. Grasp a dumbbell in each hand (or the ends of a resistance band that runs underneath your back and shoulder blades).

3. Hold your arms out to your sides with the elbows mostly straight.

4. Keeping your arms relatively straight (with soft elbows, not locked out), bring your arms together in front of your chest.

5. Hold this position for a moment and then return slowly to start. This completes 1 repetition.

6. If you're at the gym, you can make this exercise more challenging by changing the incline of the bench to vary the way you contract your muscles.

Safety Pointer: Don't allow your arms to overextend in the starting position.

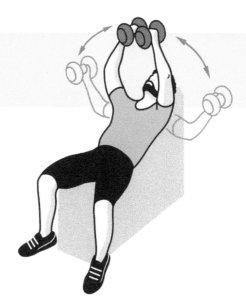

SEATED CHEST PRESS – Machine Exercise (Gym)

Muscle Groups: Chest, shoulders, triceps

1. Start by sitting on the seated chest press machine. If you're at home, you can modify this exercise by using dumbbells and lying on the floor.

2. Adjust the seat height so that your hands are in front of your shoulders.

3. Pin your shoulders back against the bench as your press the weight and move it forward gradually, extending your arms.

4. In a controlled manner, allow the weight to come back toward you by bending your arms until you've returned to starting position. This completes 1 repetition.

Safety Pointers: Always keep your shoulders pinned back as you perform the movement. Do not allow your shoulders to roll forward at any time.

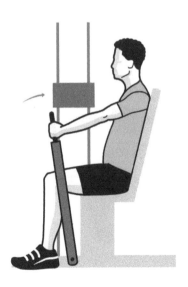 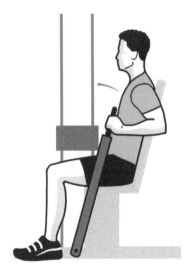

PEC DEC CHEST FLY MACHINE – Machine Exercise (Gym)

Muscle Group: Chest

1. Start by sitting on the machine with your back against the pad.

2. Grip the handles with each hand, one on each side of your body.

3. Keeping your arms somewhat straight, move the handles toward the front and center of your body until your hands meet.

4. Pause and slowly return to starting position with your arms outstretched to your sides. This completes 1 repetition.

Safety Pointers: Adjust the arms on the machine so that your chest and shoulders have just a slight stretch in the beginning of the movement. Do not start the exercise with your arms too far back, as this can put strain on the shoulder girdle and lead to injury.

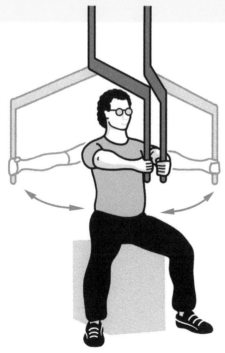

Shoulders

A complex joint, the shoulder is composed of bones, muscles, ligaments, and tendons, including the collarbones, rotator cuff muscles, shoulder blades, and upper arms. Your shoulder allows your arms to move in any plane: forward, backward, sideways, and so on. Strengthening your shoulders is a worthwhile goal, because they support many other movements.

DUMBBELL LATERAL SHOULDER RAISE – Weight Lifting Exercise (Home or Gym)

Muscle Group: Shoulders

1. Start by standing with your feet about shoulder width apart.

2. Grasp a dumbbell in each hand with your palms facing your body.

3. Keep a very slight bend in your elbows, making sure you don't lock them out.

4. Lift your arms up and out to your sides until they are about parallel to the floor.

5. Pause at the top of the motion and then lower the weights slowly back down to your sides. This completes 1 repetition.

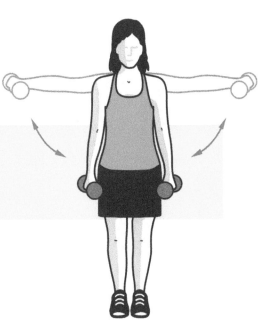

Safety Pointer: Keep a slight bend in your elbows so that your shoulders, not your arms, do the work.

DUMBBELL OVERHEAD PRESS – Weight Lifting Exercise (Home or Gym)

Muscle Group: Shoulders

1. Start by standing with your feet about shoulder width apart, keeping your abdominal core tight.

2. Grasp a dumbbell in each hand and raise your arms to bring the dumbbells up next to your ears. Your arms should be bent at the elbows making two right angles, and the ends of the dumbbell in each fist should be pointing toward your body. This is the starting position of the exercise.

3. Straighten your arms and push the dumbbells up over your head.

4. Bring your arms down into the starting position. This completes 1 repetition.

Safety Pointer: If you have a shoulder injury, do this slowly and use lighter weights or do the press one arm at a time.

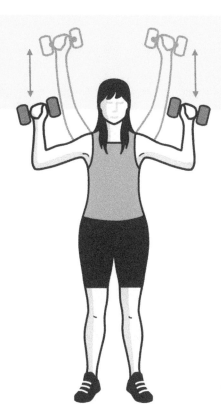

BANDED OVERHEAD SHOULDER PRESS – Banded Exercise
(Home or Gym)

Muscle Group: Shoulders

1. Start by standing with your feet about shoulder width apart.

2. Hold the band like a jump rope and step onto the middle of it with both feet. Bring your arms up next to your ears and bend at the elbow so that they form two right angles on either side of your body. This is the starting position.

3. Press your hands upward with palms facing forward until your arms straighten above your head.

4. Slowly lower your hands and bend your arms until you've resumed the starting position. This completes 1 repetition.

Safety Pointer: If the tension is too intense, try stepping on the band with one foot to give the band a little more slack.

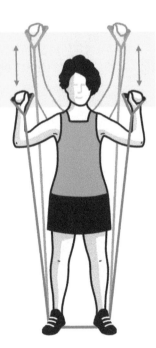

SHOULDER PRESS MACHINE – Machine Exercise (Gym)

Muscle Group: Shoulders

1. Start by sitting on the machine and placing your hands on the handles, which should be near your ears on either side of your head.

2. Using your shoulder muscles, push the handles upward.

3. Slowly return the handles to starting position to complete 1 repetition.

Safety Pointer: Before you begin, ensure your seat is the right height. Your hands should be approximately ear level when gripping the handles at the beginning of the movement.

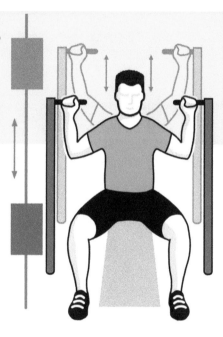

LATERAL SHOULDER RAISE MACHINE – Machine Exercise (Gym)

Muscle Group: Shoulders

1. Choose the most comfortable position for you, either sitting with your back to the machine or sitting on the machine facing the seat back.

2. Your upper arms should be next to the two moveable pads with your arms bent and your elbows by your sides.

3. Using your shoulder muscles, lift your elbows up and out to the sides.

4. Pause for a moment at the top of the movement before lowering the weight back down to your sides. This completes 1 repetition.

Safety Pointer: Make sure your elbows stay in line with your shoulders throughout the movement.

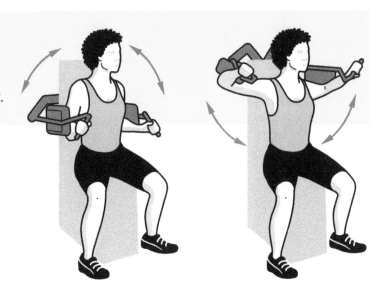

Biceps

Your biceps are in the front of your arms and are made up of the long head and the short head. The biceps tendons connect the muscles to both the shoulder joints and to the forearms. Biceps are activated through a pulling type of motion and help you to bend your arms.

DUMBBELL HAMMER CURLS – Weight Lifting Exercise (Home or Gym)

Muscle Group: Biceps

1. Start by holding a dumbbell in each hand, with your arms straight down by your sides and your palms facing inward toward the sides of your body. You can sit or stand for this exercise depending on your preference.

2. Bend your elbow to lift the dumbbell up toward your upper body, bringing the end of the dumbbell up to your lower shoulder area. You can lift one arm at a time (in an alternating fashion) or both arms together.

3. Slowly lower the weight back to the starting position. If you're alternating, repeat the same movement using the other arm. This completes 1 repetition.

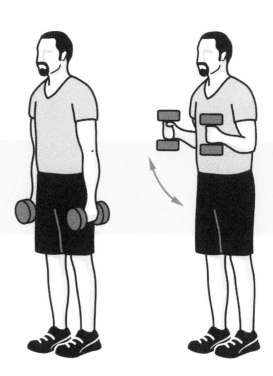

Safety Pointer: Keep your elbows tucked to your sides throughout the movement.

STANDING BANDED BICEPS CURL – Banded Exercise (Home or Gym)

Muscle Group: Biceps

1. Start by placing a resistance band under both feet and grasping both ends of the band, one end in each hand. Alternatively, hold a dumbbell in each hand if you prefer added weight.

2. With your palms facing forward, bend at the elbows slightly. This is the starting position.

3. Lift your hands up toward your shoulders, squeezing your biceps.

4. Slowly lower your arms as you release tension from the band until you return to the starting position. This completes 1 repetition.

Safety Pointers: Keep your hands in line with your elbows and shoulders as you lift the band. Always stay in control of the band as you move through the exercises by making sure the band has the right amount of tension. If you're struggling to complete a set, switch out your band for one with a looser resistance or use lighter weight dumbbells.

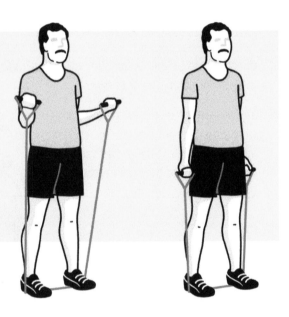

PREACHER CURL – Weight Lifting or Machine Exercise (Gym)

Muscle Group: Biceps

1. Start by sitting on the preacher curl machine with your upper arms on the inclined platform. Your chest will be next to the back of the platform as you perform the exercise while your upper arms are supported by the platform.

2. Grasp a barbell in both hands or a dumbbell in each hand. With your palms facing you, bend your elbow and use your biceps to bring the weight up to your shoulder area.

3. Slowly lower the weight back to starting position.

4. If you're using dumbbells, switch to the opposite side to duplicate the exercise. This completes 1 repetition.

> **Safety Pointers:** When using the Preacher Curl machine, don't rely on the machine's tension to move the weight back to the starting position. If you find that you're letting the machine's recoil help you complete the rep, lower the resistance to a lower weight. On the other hand, if you're able to lift the weight with so little trouble that it clanks the top of the machine, make the weight heavier.

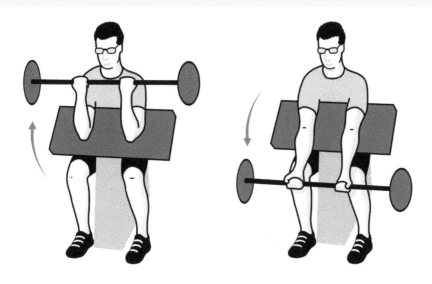

Triceps

Your triceps are formed by three muscles: the medial head, the lateral head, and the long head. Located at the rear portion of your upper arms, these muscles help you to straighten your arms by unbending and extending at the elbow.

TRICEPS DIP – Body-Weight Exercise (Home or Gym)

Muscle Group: Triceps

1. Sit on a bench or stable chair with your feet together.

2. Place your hands on the front edge of the bench or chair, palms down, next to your legs.

3. Scoot forward until your hips come off the edge and you're supported by your straight arms.

4. Bend at the elbows to slowly lower your body toward the floor. Your elbows should bend to approximately a 90-degree angle. Once you reach this angle, use your triceps to push you upward as you straighten your arms.

Safety Pointer: When doing this exercise, be sure that you don't dip to lower than a 90-degree elbow bend, as it can put excessive pressure on the shoulder and elbow joints, causing potential injury.

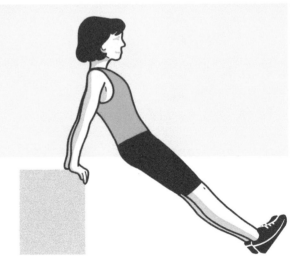

DUMBBELL KICKBACK – Weight Lifting Exercise (Home or Gym)

Muscle Group: Triceps

1. Begin by standing with your feet about shoulder width apart for even balance.

2. Grasp a dumbbell in your right hand, with your palm facing your body.

3. Step forward with your left foot and lean over, placing your left hand near your left knee for balance.

4. Bend your right elbow and bring your upper arm parallel to the floor. This is the starting position.

5. Using your right arm, raise the weight up and kick it back slowly until your arm is straight behind you.

6. Squeeze the triceps at the top of the movement and lower in a slow and controlled motion. This completes 1 repetition.

7. Finish all repetitions on one side before switching arms and repeating the process.

Safety Pointer: As you do this exercise, keep your abdominals tight to help you stabilize your body and properly focus on working just the triceps muscle.

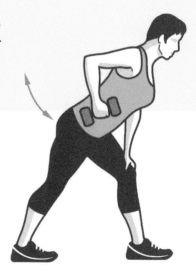

BANDED TRICEPS EXTENSION – Band Exercise (Home or Gym)

Muscle Group: Triceps

1. Step on a resistance band with both feet and grasp one end of the band in each hand. Keep your palms facing your body. Your feet should be about shoulder width apart.

2. Bend at the hips so that your torso is as close to parallel to the ground as possible.

3. Bend your elbows and bring your upper arms and elbows up, tucking them at your sides. This is the starting position.

4. Using one arm at a time, push your hand backward to straighten your arm until it, too, is parallel to the floor.

5. Squeeze your triceps muscles for a moment and then slowly bend at the elbow again, lowering your hand toward your hips. This completes 1 repetition.

Safety Pointer: For added stability, put your left knee on a bench while you work your right arm and switch when you work out the other side.

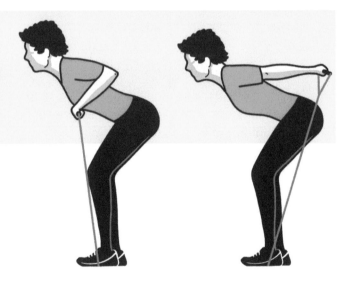

TRICEPS CABLE PUSHDOWN – Machine Exercise (Gym)

Muscle Group: Triceps

1. Start by standing in front of a cable machine with a triceps pushdown attachment. This is generally either a short bar or a double rope.

2. Grab the bar or rope on each side, ensuring you are close enough to the cable so that your upper arms will stay close to your body throughout the movement.

3. Using your triceps muscles, push the weight straight down to the ground, flexing your triceps as you do so.

4. Hold the squeeze for a moment at the bottom of the movement.

5. Let the weight come back up slowly as you bend your elbows. This completes 1 repetition.

Safety Pointers: As you complete this exercise, always keep your elbows tucked into your sides. Only the lower portion of your arms should move while your upper arms remain still.

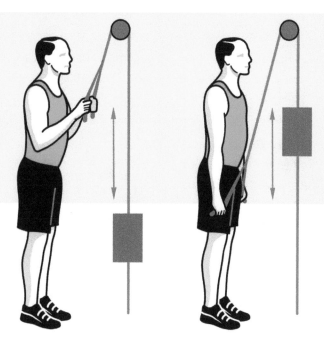

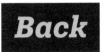

Back

Your back encompasses the rear half of your torso and extends from your neck and shoulders all the way down to your hip and gluteus areas. In addition to supporting your spine and trunk, it also assists with moving the other parts of your body that allow you to bend, twist, and more. Your back is activated and strengthened through pulling motions.

SUPERMAN – Body-Weight Exercise (Home or Gym)

Muscle Group: Back

1. Lie facedown on a mat with your arms and legs stretched out.

2. Keep your head in a neutral position resting on the mat.

3. By squeezing your back muscles, simultaneously lift your arms and legs a few inches off the ground.

4. Hold this position for a few moments before releasing your arms and legs back into a relaxed position on the ground. This completes 1 repetition.

Safety Pointer:
Remember to keep your head in a neutral position throughout this exercise as you don't want to strain your neck muscles.

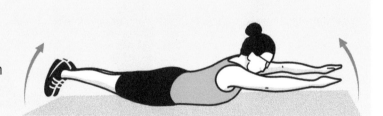

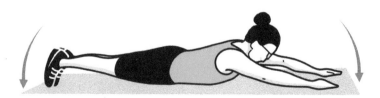

BACK

BENT-OVER DUMBBELL ROW – Weight Lifting Exercise (Home or Gym)

Muscle Group: Back

1. Start by standing with your feet about shoulder width apart.

2. Grasp a dumbbell in each hand, making sure your palms face your body.

3. Bend forward at the waist at about a 45-degree angle and allow your arms to hang down, fully extended. This is the starting position.

4. Keeping your elbows tucked close to your body, squeeze the muscles in your back as you lift the weights by bending at the elbows to bring your upper arms up and the weights by your sides.

5. Hold the squeeze for a moment before allowing the weights to return to start. Always control the descent of the weights, ensuring the descent is slow and controlled. This completes 1 repetition.

Safety Pointer: If you've suffered from any kind of back injury in the past, perform this exercise by working out one side of the body at a time while resting the other leg on a bench. This will keep you more balanced and stabilized throughout the movement.

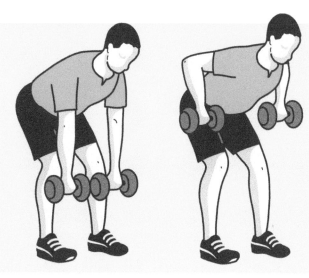

BANDED SEATED ROW – Band Exercise (Home or Gym)

Muscle Group: Back

1. Start by sitting on the floor with your legs straight in front of you.

2. Wrap a band around the bottom of both feet and grab an end in each hand.

3. Sit up straight and bend at the elbows, pulling your hands back toward your sides. Keep your elbows close to your body at all times.

4. Release the weight back to starting position slowly, controlling it the entire time. This completes 1 repetition.

Safety Pointer: Make sure to sit up straight with a slight arch in your back as you perform this exercise. This will ensure you're working your upper back muscles without straining your lower back.

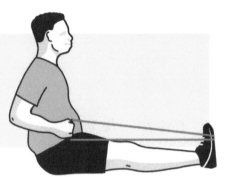

PULL APARTS – Band Exercise (Home or Gym)

Muscle Groups: Back, rear shoulders

1. Start by standing with your feet about shoulder width apart.

2. Grasp a band at each end. You may need to adjust the tension by moving your hands closer together on the band. This makes the exercise harder by putting more tension on the band.

3. Bring the band up to about chest level with your hands in front of your arms, keeping them relatively straight with a slight bend in the elbow.

4. Pull the band apart by moving your arms out to your sides and squeezing your shoulder blades together.

5. Hold the contraction for a few moments before allowing the band to return to front in a controlled motion. This completes 1 repetition.

Safety Pointer: Use a band that has a strong amount of tension, but not so much that your back and shoulders feel strained. The idea is to work the back muscles by forcing them to contract, not to recruit other nearby muscles to take over the work.

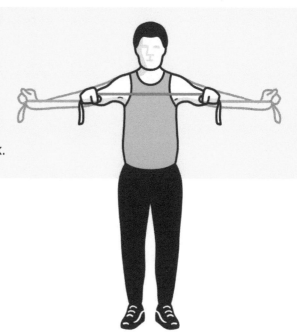

BANDED BENT-OVER ROWS – Band Exercise (Home or Gym)

Muscle Group: Back

1. Start by placing the band under both of your feet, which should be about shoulder width apart.

2. Bend at the waist, keeping your back straight while grasping the band at each end. This is the starting position.

3. Bend your elbows to bring your arms up and back until your hands are by your sides.

4. Hold the contraction for a few moments before allowing the band to move back to starting position. This completes 1 repetition.

Safety Pointer: Be sure to keep your head in line with your body and in a neutral position to prevent neck and back strain.

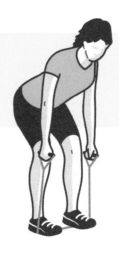
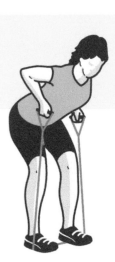

LAT PULLDOWN – Machine Exercise (Gym)

Muscle Group: Back

1. Start by sitting on a pulldown machine and facing the apparatus.

2. Reach up and grab the handles or bar with both hands, making sure that your palms are facing forward. Your arms will be outstretched above you. This is the starting position.

3. Pull downward, bringing your elbows back as you bring the weight down to the upper portion of your chest. Envision trying to touch your shoulder blades together in the back.

4. Squeeze your back muscles and then slowly allow the weight to return upward to the starting position, controlling the ascent. This completes 1 repetition.

Safety Pointers: Keep your abdominal core tight and your head in a neutral position. Stick with pulldowns in front of your head (versus behind) to protect your shoulders and avoid strain.

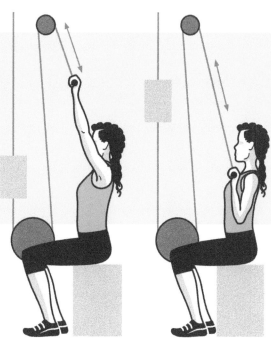

SEATED CABLE ROW – Machine Exercise (Gym)

Muscle Groups: Back, core

1. Start by sitting on the bench and leaning forward to grab the bar or handles. Your legs should be extended with your feet on the pad in front of you.

2. Pull the handles far enough back so that you can sit up straight with your arms extended in front of you. This is the starting position.

3. Pull the weight back by bending your elbows and contracting the muscles in your back. Envision trying to touch your shoulder blades together in the back.

4. Squeeze your back muscles and then slowly allow the weight to return forward to the starting position, controlling the movement. This completes 1 repetition.

Safety Pointers: As you perform this movement, keep your back from rounding forward or arching backward too far. Focus on pulling with your back muscles, not your arms.

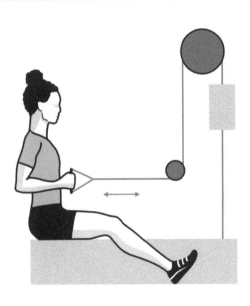 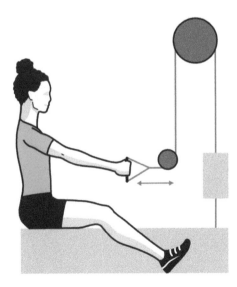

PULL-UPS – Body-Weight Exercise (Home or Gym)

Muscle Groups: Back, biceps

1. Start by placing your hands on a pull-up bar above you, palms forward.

2. Squeeze your back muscles as you bring your elbows back to move your chest upward toward the bar.

3. Once your head is past the height of the bar, let yourself return slowly to start position, controlling the rate of speed of your descent.

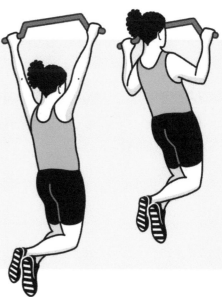

Safety Pointers: Many fitness facilities will have an assisted pull-up machine that provides a reliable place to start until you get strong enough to do pull-ups on your own. You can also get stronger by starting at the top of the pull-up movement, letting yourself down slowly, and then hanging in the outstretched position for a minute or so. Most people start this way as pull-ups require quite a bit of strength.

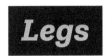

Legs

Your legs are made up of many muscles, but in general, you will work the following:

Quadriceps: The quadriceps muscle is made up of four muscles in your front thigh that help you straighten your legs and move your hips.

Hamstrings: Located at the back of your legs, hamstrings help you bend your knee and rotate your hips.

Gluteus: These muscles make up your buttocks and help your move your legs and hips.

Adductors: These are your inner thigh muscles.

Abductors: These are your outer thigh muscles.

Calves: These muscles comprise the lower portion of your legs and help you bend and flex your feet and ankles.

SQUAT – Body-Weight Exercise (Home or Gym)

Muscle Group: Legs

1. Start by standing with your feet about shoulder width apart, and your toes out at a very slight angle.

2. Place your hands on your hips (or wherever they are most comfortable).

3. Bend at the knees and simultaneously push your hips back as you squat down. Envision sitting down on a chair.

4. Push your body back up into standing position by straightening your legs and pushing upward through your heels. This completes 1 repetition.

Safety Pointer: Keep your head neutral and don't squat past a 90-degree bend in your knees.

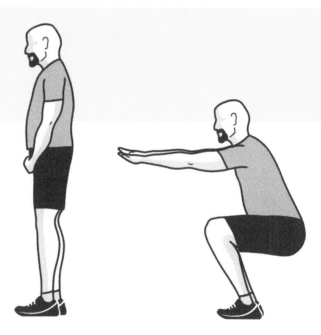

GLUTE BRIDGE – Body-Weight Exercise (Home or Gym)

Muscle Groups: Glutes, legs, core

1. Start by lying on your back on the floor or a mat with your knees bent, feet flat, and your arms by your sides.

2. Lift your hips upward off the floor or mat until you can't go any higher, squeezing your glutes hard at the top of the movement.

3. Lower your hips back down to the floor or mat. This completes 1 repetition.

Safety Pointer: Keep your head neutral and relaxed to prevent neck and back strain.

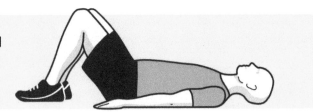

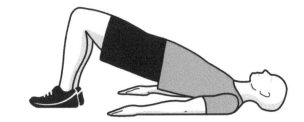

DUMBBELL SQUAT – Weight Lifting Exercise (Home or Gym)

Muscle Groups: Legs, core

1. Start by standing with your feet about shoulder width apart. Your feet should point ever so slightly outward.

2. Grasp a dumbbell in each hand, bend your arms, and bring them up near your ears. This is your starting position.

3. Move your hips backward (as if you're going to sit on a chair) as you bend your knees and lower your body toward the ground.

4. Stop when your thighs are parallel to the ground.

5. Push back up through your heels until you've returned to your starting position. This completes 1 repetition.

Safety Pointer: Keep your head neutral and don't squat past a 90-degree bend in your knees.

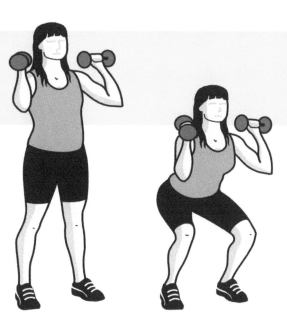

WALKING LUNGE – Body-Weight Exercise (Home or Gym)

Muscle Groups: Legs, core

1. Start by standing with your feet together and your hands on your hips.

2. Take a step forward with your left leg and bend at the knee until your thigh is parallel to the ground.

3. Push through the heel of your left foot to propel your body forward and back into upright position.

4. Repeat this movement using your opposite leg. This completes 1 repetition.

5. To make this exercise more challenging, try holding a small dumbbell in each hand as you do each lunge.

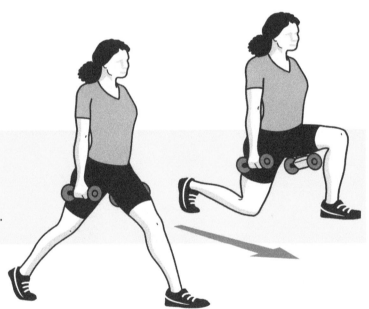

Safety Pointer: To avoid knee joint strain, don't allow your knees to pass your toes at any point.

STABILITY BALL HAMSTRING ROLL-IN – Stability Ball Exercise (Home or Gym)

Muscle Groups: Hamstrings, core

1. Start by lying on your back on a mat while resting your heels on top of a stability ball. Keep your legs straight—this is your starting position.

2. Contract your hamstrings and pull the ball toward your buttocks with your heels.

3. Using your heels, roll the ball back away from your body until your legs are fully straightened, controlling your movement slowly and evenly. This completes 1 repetition.

Safety Pointers: When your legs are extended, your body should form a straight line. Make sure to keep your hips and torso off the ground to protect your back.

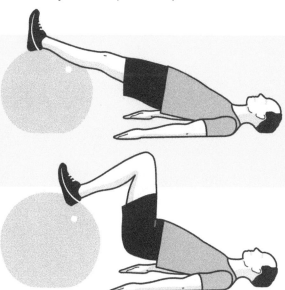

ROMANIAN DEADLIFT – Band or Weight Lifting Exercise (Home or Gym)

Muscle Groups: Hamstrings, glutes

1. Start by standing on a resistance band with both feet while holding each end in your hands. Alternately, you can hold a dumbbell in each hand. Your feet should be about shoulder width apart.

2. Float your hips back until your back is flat and parallel to the floor. Your arms will be straight down near your knees. This is your starting position.

3. Using your hamstrings and glutes, push your hips forward and your torso upward until you're fully upright. Slowly return to your starting position. This completes 1 repetition.

Safety Pointer: Allow for a very slight bend in the knees as you do this movement. You don't want to "lock out" your knees as this can put undue pressure on your joints.

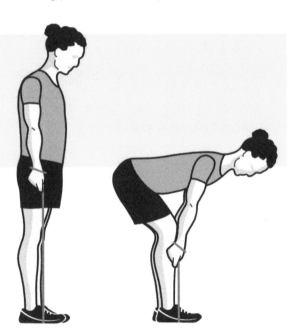

LEG PRESS – Machine Exercise (Gym)

Muscle Group: Legs

1. Start by sitting on the leg press machine with your back against the pad and your feet on the platform.

2. Adjust the seat so that when you are in your starting position, your legs are straight (always leave a very slight bend in the knee to protect your joints). Your feet should be about shoulder width apart, but you can alternate where you put your feet in order to work different areas of the legs. For example, a high and wide foot placement targets the glutes; a middle and more narrow foot placement targets the quads.

3. Release the safety on the machine and slowly lower the weight toward your chest by bending your knees until they are at a 90-degree angle.

4. Push the weight back up by pushing through your heels until your legs are straightened and you are back at starting position. This completes 1 repetition.

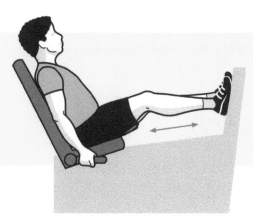

Safety Pointer: Don't allow your knees to bend past a 90-degree angle, as this can cause too much pressure on your knees and lower back.

HAMSTRING CURL – Machine Exercise (Gym)

Muscle Group: Legs

1. Start by sitting on the hamstring curl machine and adjusting the seat so that your knees are bent at a 90-degree angle. This is your starting position.

2. Push through your heels and straighten your legs to move the platform forward. (On some machines the seat will move backward instead.)

3. Control the weight by slowly bending your knees until you return to the starting position. This completes 1 repetition.

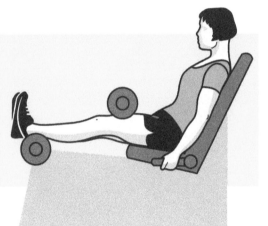

Safety Pointers: Change your foot placement to accommodate any leg injuries. To work more of your glutes, place your feet wider on the pad. To work more of the front of your legs (the quads), keep your feet closer together toward the middle of the pad.

Calves

Your calves are formed by two muscles, the gastrocnemius and the soleus. Both muscles start behind the knee and end at the Achilles tendon. Your calves help you walk, run, and jump, as well as provide stability and balance for your foot, ankle, and whole body. Calves are an important part of a full leg workout, and can often be worked on the same equipment as legs.

SEATED DUMBBELL CALF RAISE – Weight Lifting Exercise (Home or Gym)

Muscle Group: Calves

1. Start by sitting on a bench or a chair with a dumbbell in each hand. You can place something (a block or a book) under your toes to increase the range of motion during this exercise for added benefit.

2. Rest the dumbbells on your knees. This is your starting position.

3. Using your calves, raise your heels off the ground or block and squeeze your calves.

4. Slowly return to the starting position, or if your toes are on a block, enjoy an extra stretch as your heels drop past parallel. This completes 1 repetition.

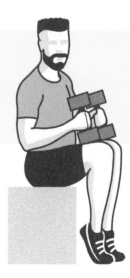

Safety Pointer: If you're using some type of platform to raise your toes, make sure you only dip down just past parallel until you feel a gentle stretch. Going farther is not necessarily better.

STANDING BANDED CALF RAISE – Band Exercise (Home or Gym)

Muscle Group: Calves

1. Start by standing on a resistance band with both feet, placing it just underneath your toes. Keeping your arms straight, grab each end of the band with your hands. This is your starting position.

2. Lift yourself up onto your toes by squeezing your calf muscles.

3. Lower yourself back to the starting position slowly while resisting the tension from the band. Make sure you feel resistance as you do this movement. If you don't, then simply wrap the band around your hands a few times to increase the tension. This completes 1 repetition.

Safety Pointer: Complete this exercise on a flat surface, otherwise it can be difficult to stabilize yourself.

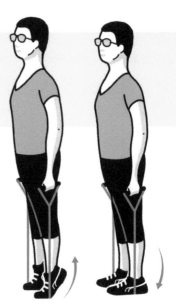

LEG PRESS CALF RAISE – Machine Exercise (Gym)

Muscle Group: Calves

1. Using the leg press machine, start by sitting with your back against the pad and your feet on the bottom edge of the platform, while keeping your toes together and the rest of your foot off the edge. This is your starting position.

2. Push forward on the platform with your toes (squeezing your calves) to mimic the movement of standing on your toes.

3. Slowly return the weight to starting position and allow yourself to feel a deep stretch through your calves. This completes 1 repetition.

Safety Pointer: Always keep a slight bend in your knees as you do this movement to reduce stress and pressure on the knee joint.

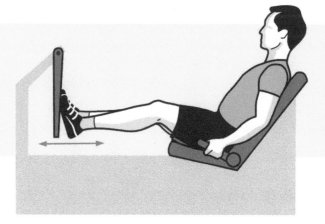

Abdominals

Your abdominals are in the front midsection of your body and help support your skeletal structure, protect your internal organs, and move your body. There are four main areas of the abs: the rectus abdominus; the internal and external obliques; and the hidden layer of muscle, the transversus abdominus, that wraps around your core for support.

PLANK – Body-Weight Exercise (Home or Gym)

Muscle Groups: Abdominals and core

1. Start on all fours, with your hands and knees on a mat.

2. Shift onto your forearms so that your elbows are directly beneath your shoulders.

3. Straighten your legs and get up onto your toes so that the only parts of your body that are touching the floor are your forearms and your toes.

4. Maintain this hold for as long as you can. Try starting with 20 seconds and work your way up to two minutes.

Safety Pointer: Keep your body in a straight line and keep your head in a neutral position. Your hips should be tucked and your abdominal core tight.

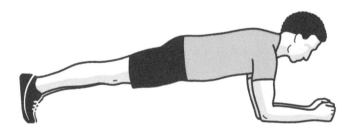

CRUNCH – Body-Weight Exercise (Home or Gym)

Muscle Group: Abdominals

1. Start by lying on your back with your knees bent and your feet flat on the floor.

2. Place your arms behind your head and lift yourself off the floor ever so slightly. This is your starting position.

3. Look straight up toward the ceiling and lift your head and shoulders up and off the floor.

4. Hold this "crunch" position for a moment before returning to your starting position. This completes 1 repetition.

Safety Pointers: Be careful not to pull your head and neck too far *forward*. Only move your head and upper body *upward*, so as not to strain your beck or back.

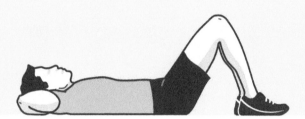

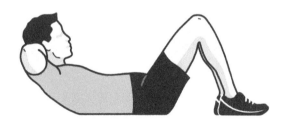

STABILITY BALL KNEE-INS – Stability Ball Exercise (Home or Gym)

Muscle Groups: Abdominals, upper body

1. Begin by placing the tops of your feet on a stability ball and your hands flat on the ground in front of you, keeping your arms straight. (You'll be in a regular push-up position, but with the tops of your feet on the ball.)

2. Pull the ball toward your chest by bending your knees. Your feet will help guide the movement, but make sure you're using your abs to complete the exercise.

3. Push your feet away from your chest and slowly straighten your legs. This completes 1 repetition.

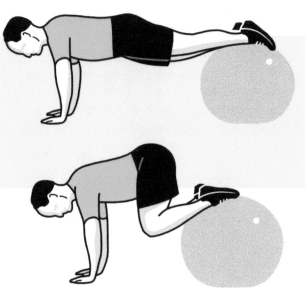

Safety Pointer: This is a more advanced exercise, so ensure that you can hold a plank exercise for 30 to 60 seconds before attempting this. Avoid it if you have shoulder issues or injuries.

HANGING LEG RAISES – Machine Exercise (Gym)

Muscle Groups: Abdominals, upper body

1. Start by standing in the captain's chair and placing your forearms on the pads. Grasp the handles in each hand. This is your starting position.

2. Lift your feet off the sides of the chair as you bend your knees slightly and bring your thighs up toward your chest.

3. Slowly lower your knees back down toward the ground as you straighten your legs. This completes 1 repetition.

Safety Pointer: If you have shoulder issues or injuries, avoid this exercise because it requires considerable upper-body strength to do this movement.

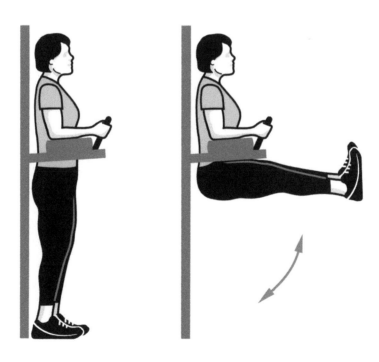

6

FLEXIBILITY TRAINING

In this chapter, you'll learn why flexibility is important, and how you can cultivate and maintain it as you get older. You'll also learn how to perform each flexibility exercise properly so that you can get the most out of your workouts as you work your way through the six-week workout plan.

Why Flexibility Training?

Flexibility training is an important component of a well-rounded workout program. According to the National Strength and Conditioning Association (NSCA), flexibility training is a fundamental aspect of a good training regimen because being able to move freely through a full range of motion can help you perform better when exercising as well as when doing everyday activities.

The NSCA also stresses the importance of flexibility when it comes to avoiding and preventing injuries. Just because stretching doesn't directly improve strength or cardiovascular conditioning doesn't mean it's not as important as other types of exercise. Although it's common to leave stretching exercises until the end of a workout, stretching should ideally be done before *and* after getting into your other routines to help prevent injuries from happening.

How Much Do I Need?

According to the American College of Sports Medicine (ACSM), healthy adults should engage in a stretching program at a minimum of two to three times per week. They recommend spending a full minute on each stretch, even if you break them up into shorter lengths of time. If you can only hold a stretch for 15 seconds, consider repeating that stretch three more times to fulfill your full minute of stretching for that area.

The ACSM also notes that it's important to include stretches for all the main muscle and tendon groups, so ideally aim to fit these stretches into your fitness program at least three times a week:

→ Neck
→ Shoulders
→ Chest
→ Torso
→ Lower back
→ Hips
→ Legs (both the quads in front and the hamstrings in back)
→ Calves
→ Ankles

Making Progress

Making progress with your flexibility means challenging yourself during each workout, mindfully altering something each time to make it a little more difficult and rewarding in turn.

When it comes to flexibility, there are dynamic and static stretches. Dynamic stretches use muscles to produce the stretch by putting the muscles and joints through a full range of motion. Dynamic stretches involve movement, like swinging your leg back and forth like a pendulum in preparation for a jog or doing arm circles before a swimming session.

Static stretches are stretches that you hold. Imagine stretching your hamstrings by placing your leg on a platform in front of you and leaning forward over that leg. You could easily do this in between exercise sets and after your workout, once your muscles are warmed up and limber.

You can mix up your flexibility workout by include things like yoga and Tai Chi, which improve flexibility and bring other benefits like relieving stress, boosting mood, helping increase circulation, strengthening muscles, improving balance, and much more.

HEALTH CONCERNS

It's always best to consult your physician or physical therapist before starting a new flexibility program. Depending on your medical history, they may suggest modifications to common exercises or want you to use caution when stretching certain areas of your body.

When stretching, remember not to stretch a "cold" muscle, so gently warm up your muscles first with a brisk walk, jumping jacks, or body squats—whatever it takes to get your circulation moving. Or you can stretch after a full workout as a cool-down session. Stretching immediately after your workout is almost always a safe bet as your body should be fully warmed up and your muscles will be receptive to both dynamic and static stretching movements.

Finally, beware of bouncing when you're performing a static stretch. You should get into the stretched position and hold it. It's okay to lean into the stretch during the hold to make it more challenging, just avoid the bounce.

Flexibility Exercises

Before beginning your flexibility training, start with 5 to 10 minutes of walking, jogging, using the elliptical, jumping rope, or another activity that gets your heart rate up safely. You can also start with myofascial release, employing foam rollers and other similar tools like foam balls and handheld rollers to help work out the knots in your muscles.

To do so, simply roll the affected area on the foam roller or on the ball. As you gently roll your body, the applied pressure helps to "release" muscle knots, allowing for a more effective stretching session. Note that it's important to address both stability joints (knees, lower back) and movement joints (shoulders, hips, middle spine) when stretching.

Consider including dynamic stretches that cover these main patterns of movement:

→ Bending and lifting motions
→ Single-leg movements
→ Pulling motions
→ Twisting movements

To improve your flexibility overall, address all the muscles in your body when you stretch, and mix it up if you like! While you don't need to stretch every area every single day, it's a good idea to stretch the areas you're going to be using later.

Remember, dynamic stretches use movement and are designed to help your body get primed for a specific exercise or sport. You may want to simulate some of the movements your body will be making, like torso twists if you'll be playing baseball, softball, or golfing.

QUADRICEPS STRETCH – Body-Weight Stretch (Home or Gym)

Muscle Group: Quadriceps

1. Start by standing with your feet about shoulder width apart.

2. Pick up your right leg and bend it upward behind you so that your foot is near your glutes.

3. Grab your right foot with your right hand and gently pull it until you feel a stretch through the front of your leg. Hold the stretch for about 20 seconds. This completes 1 repetition.

4. Repeat on the opposite side for the same length of time.

Safety Pointer: If needed, stabilize yourself by holding on to a chair or placing your hand on a wall.

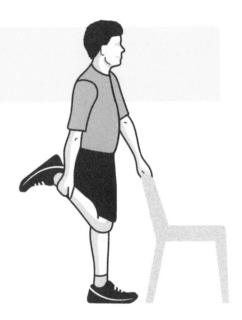

HAMSTRING STRETCH – Body-Weight Stretch (Home or Gym)

Muscle Group: Hamstrings

1. Start by standing with your feet about shoulder width apart.

2. Take your left leg and lift it, placing it on a raised platform or chair seat in front of you. Make sure to keep your leg straight (not bent at the knee).

3. Gently lean forward at the hips to bring your torso over your leg and reach toward your toes.

4. Continue moving forward until you feel a comfortable stretch through the back of your leg. Hold the stretch for a minute and then return to standing. This completes 1 repetition.

5. Repeat on the opposite leg for the same length of time.

Safety Pointer: For added stability, hold on to something like a chair or the wall as you stretch.

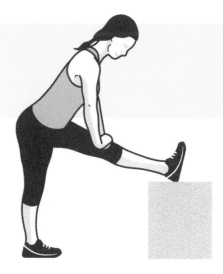

INNER-THIGH STRETCH – Body-Weight Stretch (Home or Gym)

Muscle Group: Inside thighs

1. Start by sitting on the floor with your knees bent and your feet together in front of you. Allow your knees to move out to each side.

2. Grab on to your feet and lean forward until you feel a stretch through your inner thighs.

3. Hold the stretch for a few moments and then release the tension. This completes 1 repetition.

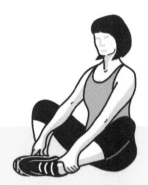

Safety Pointer: Avoid bouncing, but rest your elbows on your knees and gently push down to enhance your stretch.

CALF STRETCH – Body-Weight Stretch (Home or Gym)

Muscle Group: Calves

1. Start by standing in front of a wall.

2. Take a step backward with your left leg, then lean forward and place your hands on the wall in front of you.

3. Press your right heel into the ground as you continue to lean forward, feeling a stretch throughout your calf muscle.

4. Switch feet and do the same stretch on the other side. This completes 1 repetition.

> **Safety Pointer:** Bend your knees slightly to feel a deeper stretch through the calves.

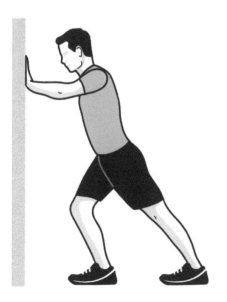 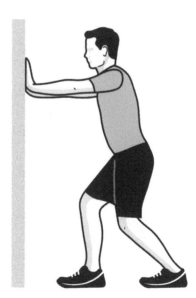

Back Stretch – Body-Weight Stretch (Home or Gym)

Muscle Group: Back

1. Start by standing a foot or two away from a wall, table, or similarly stable structure.

2. Stretch out your arms and place your hands on the surface while leaning forward at the waist.

3. Feel a gentle stretch through your back. Then, slowly roll your body up into a standing position. This completes 1 repetition.

Safety Pointer: If you have any type of shoulder injury, avoid putting your hands on a surface and simply bend at the waist and allow your torso to hang forward while you feel a comfortable stretch through your back.

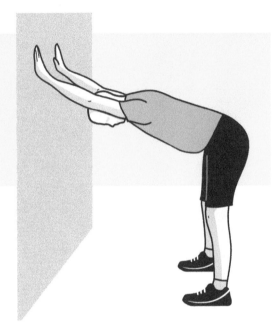

CHEST STRETCH – Body-Weight Stretch (Home or Gym)

Muscle Groups: Chest, shoulders

1. Start by standing in a doorway with your feet about shoulder width apart and placing your left forearm on the edge of the frame. Bend your arm and keep your elbow at about chest level.

2. Gently lean your torso forward until you feel a comfortable stretch across your chest area.

3. Remove your arm from the wall and repeat on the opposite side of the body. This completes 1 repetition.

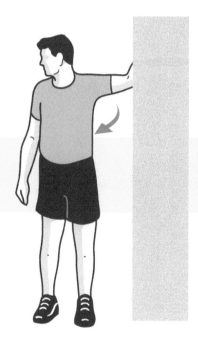

Safety Pointer: Perform the stretch slowly and avoid rotating your arm too far back.

HIP STRETCH – Body-Weight Stretch (Home or Gym)

Muscle Groups: Hips, lower back, glutes

1. Start by lying on your back with your feet flat and your knees bent.

2. Pick up your right leg and turn it so that you can place your right ankle across your left knee.

3. Reach your right arm through your legs and your left arm around the outside of your left thigh to pull your left leg toward your torso. You should feel a nice stretch through your entire hip region.

4. Place your right leg back on the floor and repeat the stretch using the left leg. This completes 1 repetition.

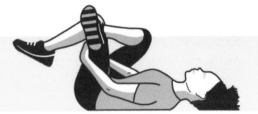

Safety Pointer: Keep your back flat and your head on the floor as you do this stretch.

OVERHEAD TRICEPS STRETCH – Body-Weight Stretch (Home or Gym)

Muscle Group: Triceps

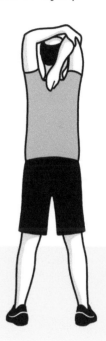

1. Start by standing with your feet about shoulder width apart. Lift your right arm up and bend at the elbow so that your hand is behind your head.

2. Using your left arm, gently grab your right elbow and pull your arm toward and slightly behind your head.

3. Feel a comfortable stretch in your right triceps muscles and then release.

4. Repeat the stretch on the left side. This completes 1 repetition.

Safety Pointer: Don't pull too hard when performing this stretch. Keep a gentle pressure on the arm being stretched but never pull so hard that you cause pain.

ARM CIRCLES – Body-Weight Stretch (Home or Gym)

Muscle Groups: Arms, shoulders

1. Start by standing with your feet about shoulder width apart.

2. Raise your arms straight out to your sides, keeping your hands fully extended. This is your starting position.

3. Rotate your arms forward in a small circle. This completes 1 repetition.

4. To complete a full set, do 10 circles in the forward direction, gradually increasing the size of the circles before switching directions, and do 10 more rotations in the opposite direction.

5. For an additional stretch, repeat the same sequence but flex your hands upward. Then repeat the sequence again with your hands flexed down.

LEG PENDULUMS – Body-Weight Stretch (Home or Gym)

Muscle Groups: Legs, hips

1. Start by standing with your feet slightly apart and your hands on your hips. For added balance and stability, grab on to a chair or a countertop.

2. Lift your right leg and swing it forward and backward. This completes 1 repetition.

3. To complete a set, perform 10 repetitions on the right side, increasing your range of motion with each leg swing. Then, switch legs and repeat the sequence.

TORSO TWISTS – Body-Weight Stretch (Home or Gym)

Muscle Groups: Back, abdominals

1. Start by standing with your feet shoulder width apart.

2. Place your hands on your hips.

3. Keep the lower half of your body facing forward while twisting your upper body and head to the right as far as is comfortable for you.

4. Bring your upper body back to center and repeat on the opposite side. This completes 1 repetition.

CAT COW – Body-Weight Stretch (Home or Gym)

Muscle Groups: Back and lower back, shoulders

1. Start by getting on your hands and knees, with your palms down and hands directly under your shoulders. Your back should be flat like a tabletop. This is your starting position.

2. Lower your head and arch your back upward (like a cat) until you feel a comfortable stretch through your upper back, shoulders, and hip area.

3. Bring your belly down and gently arch your back in the opposite direction, raising your head up and back. Feel a stretch through the front of your body. This completes 1 repetition.

4. To complete a full set, repeat both movements 10 times.

7

BALANCE TRAINING

In this chapter, you'll learn how to round out your fitness plan with balance training. We'll explore different exercises and techniques that you can use to improve your balance and stability, how to do these exercises with proper form, and how to keep your workouts fresh and interesting.

Once you have a solid grasp on the basics of balance training, you'll be able to breeze through these exercises in no time. Feel free to explore some of the other activities discussed at the end of the chapter as well, like yoga, Pilates, and Tai Chi, which provide fun ways to improve your balance solo, with a friend, or in a class setting.

Why Balance Training?

Not only does balance training engage and strengthen all the muscles of your core (which includes your abdominals and your back muscles), but training your core for balance can help you minimize the risk for other injuries as well. A weak core can contribute to other sports-related injuries. Bicyclists with a weak core, for example, can suffer back and neck pain, sometimes even requiring medical attention. When you work on strengthening your core and your balance, you increase your control over other areas of your body, like your hips and shoulder girdle. In this way, everything truly does connect to everything else.

Because balance training helps strengthen your stabilizer muscles and your core, it also improves your joint stability. Your power comes from your core, so a stronger core means an overall stronger body. Balance will help you with everyday activities as well as with physical exercise and movement. Better balance will help you avoid falls, which can become dangerous as we age. One-third of adults aged 65 and older suffer from fall-related injuries, so you can't get started too soon on balance improvement.

How Much Do I Need?

Because you use your balancing skills for virtually everything you do, from getting out of the car to picking something up from the floor, your stabilizer muscles are working overtime to keep you upright and injury-free. As a result, you really can't overdo your balance training.

Balance, autonomy, and self-confidence are all interrelated. Being consistent with your exercise program will help you focus and feel good, both mentally and physically, as you go about your daily activities. Although you can do as much balance training as you like, an effective balance-training program revolves around three to five training sessions per week, with four or more balance exercises per session.

Making Progress

Always remember to start with caution. You can progress to more challenging movements as you get stronger and are better able to balance. The longer you work at it incrementally, the more likely you'll suddenly notice one day that you're not grabbing for that countertop as often or that you can hold your leg in the air longer than you could at first.

Increasing the strength of your body, particularly your legs, through your resistance-training program will also help you boost your ability to balance, so all the effort you're putting into your resistance-training program is also paying dividends when it comes to enhanced balance.

As you progress, you may want to experiment by working with unstable surfaces, like a BOSU ball. A BOSU (an acronym for "both sides utilized" or "both sides up") ball has one flat surface (that's usually on the ground) and one that's soft and rounded, facing up. The rounded, inflated surface of the BOSU provides an unsteady surface to help challenge your balancing skills and engage your core, resulting in a stronger center and more refined balance skills all around.

Other ways to improve balance include activities like yoga, Pilates, and Tai Chi. Yoga focuses on both physical and mental balance, helping to foster the essential mind-body connection. This connection helps you to tune in to your body, feel the exercises and poses as you do them, and release emotional and physical stress. Yoga focuses on alignment (so that your body can be optimally stable), strength (to give you the ability to hold your balance), and attention (being mindful of your body and its positioning). When looking to build your balance, consider trying out Iyengar yoga or the more mainstream, popular Hatha yoga.

Pilates, founded in 1920 by Joseph Pilates, was initially designed for rehabilitation purposes. It aims to strengthen your core, improve your posture and balance, and help you stabilize your body for better overall posture. This is a mode of exercise that uses resistance training and muscle-building tactics, but it is gentle and lightweight, so it doesn't add bulk to the body or stress the joints, tendons, and ligaments.

While yoga focuses on many standing poses (which is why it's great for balance training), Pilates tends to mostly take place either on a mat or on what's called a "reformer," which is a machine designed to help you enhance your stretches. Because many Pilates stretches are done from the floor, it's naturally a more core-centric workout.

Tai Chi, or "meditation in motion," can relieve stress, cultivate a mind-body connection, build better balance, enhance strength and flexibility, increase attention and mental clarity, and improve mood and sleep. Try taking a class (in a studio or online) and see what you think!

HEALTH CONCERNS

Along with balance training comes a modicum of caution. People with injuries, such as hip or knee injuries, should use caution when working on improving their balance. You don't need to skip these exercises altogether if you are working around an injury, but always ensure that you have something you can use to steady yourself nearby, like a chair, countertop, or wall. Practice your balance for short periods until you feel stronger and more confident. Doing balance-training exercises three to five times a week for a maximum of 10 to 15 minutes at a time should be plenty to help you boost your balance.

Balance Exercises

Although it may seem simple enough compared to other types of exercises within this book, the importance of balance can't be overstated. After all, without a strong ability to balance, you can't perform even the simplest everyday movements, let alone exercises. Within this section, you'll discover some simple exercises to improve your balance using the floor, your own body weight, and a variety of optional additions like chairs, countertops, weights, aerobic steps, and BOSU balls.

TIGHTROPE WALK – Body-Weight Exercise (Home or Gym)

Muscle Groups: Arms, legs, core

1. Start by standing with your feet together and your arms up and straight out to your sides.

2. Keep your head in a neutral position and look straight ahead.

3. Pick up your right foot and place your heel in front of your left toes so that your feet form a straight line. This completes 1 repetition.

4. To complete a full set, repeat the steps with your left foot and continue your walk for as far as space allows.

5. As you get accustomed to this exercise and your balance improves, you can pause and hold your foot up for a few moments before placing it on the ground.

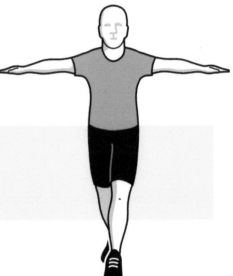

Safety Pointer: Make sure you have enough space to perform this exercise effectively without bumping or tripping over objects or furniture.

SIDE LEG RAISE – Body-Weight Exercise (Home or Gym)

Muscle Groups: Legs, core

1. Start by standing with your feet together and your hands on your hips.

2. Keep your legs straight during this exercise and your feet in a neutral stance.

3. Lift your right leg up and out to the side, keeping your foot pointed forward and your leg straight.

4. Hold your leg out to the side as long as you can before bringing it back to the starting position. Don't worry if you can't hold it out for very long at first. This exercise takes practice, and the idea is to improve over time.

5. Repeat the exercise using your opposite leg. This completes 1 repetition.

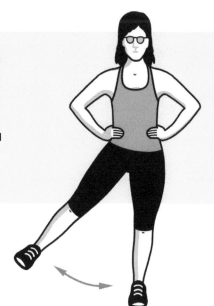

Safety Pointer: For an added challenge, try this exercise while standing on an unstable surface like a BOSU ball. But because this is significantly more difficult than standing on a flat surface, consider doing this exercise near something secure that you can grab on to if necessary, like a sturdy chair or countertop.

ONE-LEGGED STAND – Body-Weight Exercise (Home or Gym)

Muscle Groups: Legs, core

1. Start by standing with your feet together in front of a chair or a countertop that you can reach easily.

2. Grab the edge of the counter or the back of a chair for balance.

3. Lean forward slightly and lift your left foot off the ground.

4. Bend your left knee until your foot is behind you and your calf is parallel to the floor.

5. Hold this position for 10 to 15 seconds before returning your foot to the floor.

6. Repeat the exercise using your opposite leg. This completes 1 repetition.

Safety Pointers: Once you get acclimated to this exercise and your balance improves, experiment by forgoing the chair or countertop. Reduce your chances of injury by practicing for a few seconds before fully committing to the no-hands version.

WEIGHT SHIFTS – Body-Weight Exercise (Home or Gym)

Muscle Groups: Legs, core

1. Start by standing with your feet about shoulder width apart.

2. You may need to use your arms for balance if you're just starting this program. Otherwise, place your hands on your hips.

3. Lift your right leg and hold it a few inches off the ground in front of you for 30 seconds. If you need to stabilize yourself, do this exercise near a countertop or a chair.

4. Put your right foot back down on the ground and repeat the process with your left foot. This completes 1 repetition.

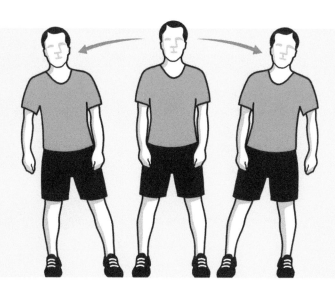

Safety Pointers:
As always, start slowly and don't be afraid to hold on to something like a chair as you get accustomed to the movement. Give yourself some grace as you work your way up to longer and more stable holds.

STANDING CRUNCH WITH UNDER-LEG CLAP – Body-Weight Exercise (Home or Gym)

Muscle Group: Legs

1. Start by standing with your feet together.

2. Pick up your right leg and lift it until your thigh is parallel to the ground.

3. Raise your arms straight above your head and clap your hands together.

4. Swing your arms all the way down under your right leg to clap your hands together again. This completes 1 repetition.

5. To complete a full set, repeat the exercise five times on one side, then switch to the opposite leg.

Safety Pointer: This may sound like a simple exercise, but it can be quite challenging. Keep close to something stable that you can reach for, if necessary.

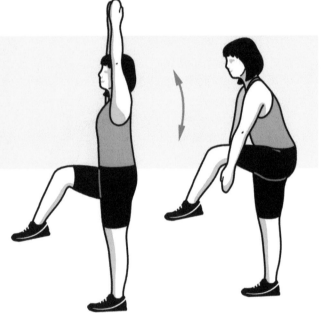

ROLLING FOREARM SIDE PLANK – Body-Weight Exercise (Home or Gym)

Muscle Groups: Abdominals, core, legs, arms

1. Start in the normal plank position by resting on your forearms with your legs straight (see page 84 for a refresher, if needed).

2. Shift your forearms so that they are folded underneath your chest (instead of facing forward).

3. Roll to your left and stack your feet to bring yourself into a side plank position.

4. Extend your right arm out and upward as your roll over onto your left forearm.

5. Hold this side position with your arm extended for a count of five.

6. Bring your right arm back down to the floor and put your weight onto your right forearm.

7. Repeat the entire sequence on your left side, then return to center. This completes 1 repetition.

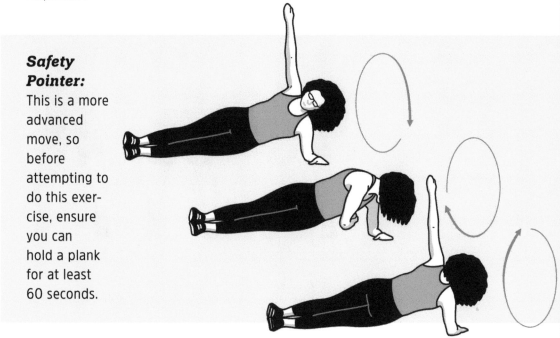

Safety Pointer: This is a more advanced move, so before attempting to do this exercise, ensure you can hold a plank for at least 60 seconds.

ARM SEQUENCE WITH LIFTED HEELS – Body-Weight Exercise (Home or Gym)

Muscle Groups: Legs, core, arms, shoulders

1. Start with your feet about shoulder width apart and your arms straight down at your sides.

2. Lift your heels off the floor a few inches so you're standing primarily on your toes.

3. Bend your arms and bring them up simultaneously into a biceps curl (see page 58 for a refresher). This is your starting position.

4. From the curl position, raise your arms straight up overhead.

5. Bring your arms back down to the starting position. This completes 1 repetition.

Safety Pointers: This exercise can be done with or without dumbbells. If you choose to use them during this movement, use light dumbbells—about 2 to 3 pounds—to avoid overstraining.

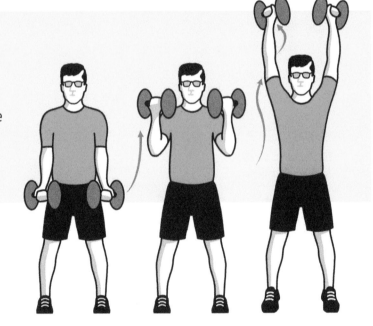

TOE TAPS – Body-Weight Exercise (Home or Gym)

Muscle Groups: Legs, calves, core

1. Start by standing with your feet about shoulder width apart in front of a platform. Ideally the platform should be at least 12 inches high, but you can use anything—a simple stair, an aerobics step, or a BOSU ball.

2. Lift your right leg and tap the platform with the ball of your foot.

3. Bring this foot back to the ground and repeat with the opposite foot. This completes 1 repetition.

4. Once you have this movement down, try pushing off from your left heel while your right foot is touching the platform and switching foot positions in the air. Speeding up your pace or touching a higher platform can make this exercise harder. Just be sure to start out slowly and work your way up to more difficult moves.

5. Pump your arms in a back-and-forth motion like you would if you were running.

6. To complete a full set, continue alternating toe taps for up to 60 seconds at a time.

Safety Pointer: Make sure to keep your eyes on the platform to stay balanced, especially as you increase your speed.

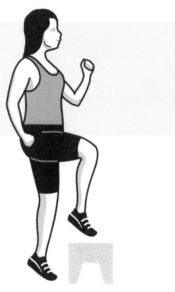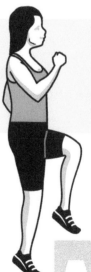

8

FIRE IT UP

It's time to put what we've learned into practice with a six-week exercise program!

For home workouts, you'll need the same equipment that you've been using for the previous workouts, namely a light set of dumbbells, some lightweight resistance bands, and a stability ball. Of course, all the exercises designed for home workouts can be completed in a fitness facility as well.

Think of these workouts as both a guide and a starting point. As you gain confidence in your routines, feel free to branch out on your own with new, more challenging, or different exercises.

When you embark on a new journey, it's important to review your goals often. Set deadlines and checkpoints for yourself along the way and check in with yourself once a week using the included weekly check-ins to document your progress and adjust your program accordingly. Always take a few moments to log your progress in a spreadsheet or workout journal. Keeping track of your workouts will go a long way toward staying motivated and reaching your goals.

Week One

"Without dreams and goals, there is no living, only merely existing, and that is not why we are here."

—Mark Twain

When it comes to starting anything new, you just need to commit to your journey. Don't worry about being perfect or getting everything aligned before you start—a phenomenon known as "paralysis by analysis." Just get started and know that we will course correct along the way. To inspire yourself as you start, try repeating an affirmation like this:

"I will get started in the direction of my goals. I am proud of myself for taking these steps forward. I will give myself grace as I learn and adjust."

WEEK ONE: HOME WORKOUT

Days of the Week: Choose 3 nonconsecutive days to work out. Make sure to have at least 1 day in between workouts so your body has time to recover and you're not doing the same exercises 2 days in a row.

Approximate Workout Time: 1 hour (including a 5-minute warm-up and a 10-minute cool-down)

Overview: A 5-minute warm-up followed by 10 minutes of balance training. Next, you'll do the resistance portion of your workout, followed by 15 minutes of endurance training, and ending with a 10-minute flexibility exercise cool-down.

Reminder: Unless otherwise noted, do 12 to 15 repetitions for all resistance exercises (this makes up 1 set). Choose a weight that starts to feel relatively heavy for you at 10 to 12 repetitions.

1 Warm-Up

Start your workout with a 5-minute warm-up such as walking, biking, jogging, and so on.

2 Balance Training

If you are just starting a workout routine, 1 run-through of these exercises should suffice. If you are more experienced, you can go through the sequence 2 or 3 times.

1. Tightrope Walk

(page 106) – Walk 20 steps in each direction.

2. Side Leg Raise

(page 107) – Do 5 leg raises on each side and repeat 2 times.

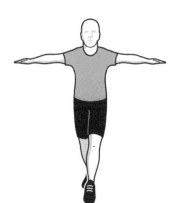

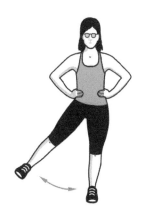

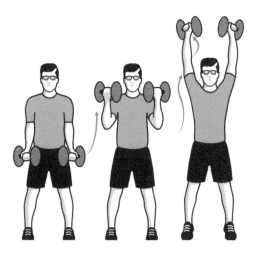

3. Arm Sequence with Lifted Heels

(page 112) – Do 10 repetitions, take a 10-second break, then do 10 more repetitions.

3 Resistance Training

1. Regular Push-Ups

(page 46) – Aim for 12 to 15 repetitions.

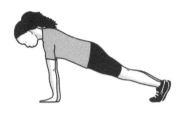

2. Dumbbell Lateral Shoulder Raise

(page 52)

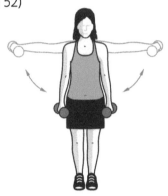

3. Standing Banded Biceps Curl

(page 58) – Do these with both arms at the same time or one arm at a time.

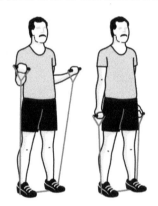

4. Triceps Dip

(page 60) – If these are difficult, keep your knees bent and don't go all the way down until you build up strength.

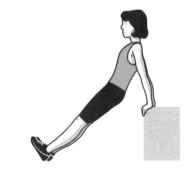

5. Superman

(page 64) – Hold for 10 to 20 seconds, repeat 3 to 5 times.

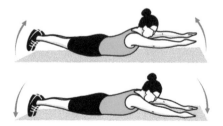

6. Squat

(page 73) – Start with 10 repetitions, then work your way up to 20.

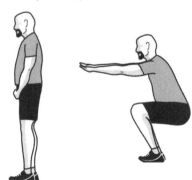

7. Standing Banded Calf Raise

(page 82) – Do 15 to 20 repetitions.

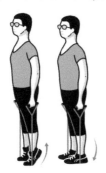

8. Plank

(page 84) – Hold this for as long as you can, aiming for 60 seconds.

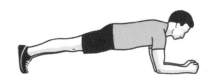

4 Endurance Training

For 15 minutes, do an endurance activity like a brisk walk, light jog, or easy bike ride.

5 Flexibility Training

Hold each stretch for a count of 10. If you have extra time, run through this sequence 2 to 3 times.

1. Quadriceps Stretch

(page 92)

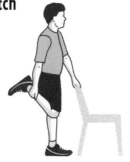

2. Hamstring Stretch

(page 93)

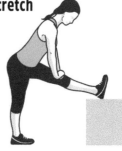

3. Chest Stretch

(page 97)

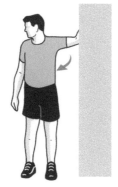

4. Back Stretch

(page 96)

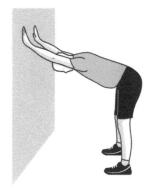

WEEK ONE: GYM WORKOUT

Days of the Week: Three nonconsecutive days

Approximate Workout Time: 1 hour (including a 5-minute warm-up and a 10-minute cool-down)

Overview: A 5-minute warm-up followed by 10 minutes of balance training. Next, you'll do the resistance portion of your workout, followed by 15 minutes of endurance training, and ending with a 10-minute flexibility exercise cool-down.

Reminder: Unless otherwise noted, do 12 to 15 repetitions for all resistance exercises. Choose a weight that starts to feel relatively heavy for you at 10 to 12 repetitions.

1 Warm-Up

Start with a gentle 5-minute warm-up. You can walk on a treadmill, ride a bicycle, do some step-ups, or whatever you like.

2 Balance Training

If you are just starting a workout routine, 1 run-through of these exercises should suffice. If you are feeling up to it, go through the sequence 2 or 3 times.

1. Tightrope Walk

(page 106) – Walk 20 steps in each direction.

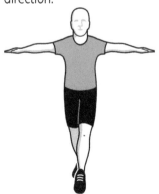

2. Side Leg Raise

(page 107) – Do 5 leg raises on each side and repeat 2 times.

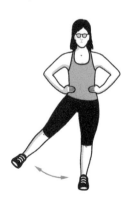

3. Arm Sequence with Lifted Heels

(page 112) – Do 10 repetitions, take a 10- to 15-second break, then do 10 more repetitions.

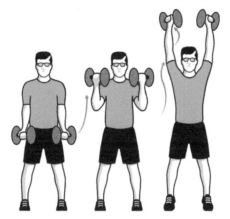

3 Resistance Training

1. Seated Chest Press

(page 50) – Do 12 to 15 repetitions, controlling the weight in both directions.

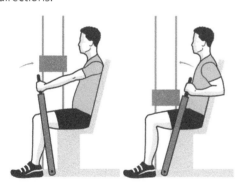

2. Dumbbell Lateral Shoulder Raise

(page 52) – Do these with both arms at the same time or one arm at a time.

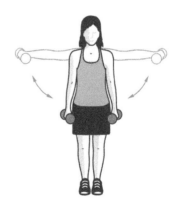

3. Triceps Dip

(page 60) – Use the edge of a bench or a machine if available.

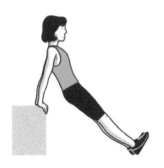

4. Seated Cable Row

(page 70) – Keep your upper body stable as you perform this movement.

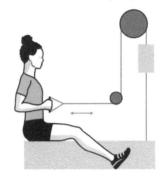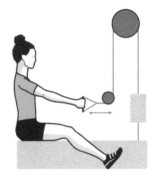

5. Squat

(page 73) – Start with 10 repetitions, then work your way up to 20.

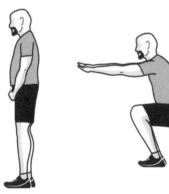

6. Seated Dumbbell Calf Raise

(page 81) – Do 15 to 20 repetitions.

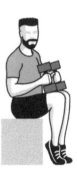

7. Plank

(page 84) – Hold this for as long as you can, aiming for 60 seconds.

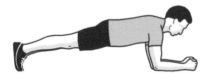

4 Endurance Training

For 15 minutes, do an activity that allows you to get slightly out of breath. Try using a stair climber, an elliptical machine, or an indoor bike.

5 Flexibility Training

Finish up and cool down with some flexibility training. Hold each stretch for a count of 10. If you have extra time, run through this sequence 2 to 3 times.

1. Quadriceps Stretch
(page 92)

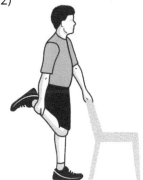

2. Hamstring Stretch
(page 93)

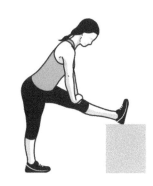

3. Chest Stretch
(page 97)

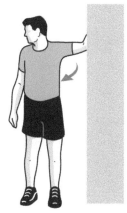

4. Back Stretch
(page 96)

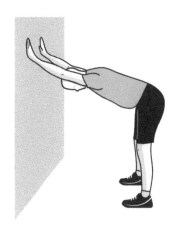

Week One: Weekly Check-In

Your week-one check-in will help you determine a starting point so that you can assess how you feel now and then come back to this page later to see how far you've come. It's exciting to witness the changes in your body, health, and mindset, so documenting it all can make it fun, interesting, and motivating.

1. How did you feel before starting the program? In what ways do you feel different now?

2. How were your nutritional choices this week? Did you make healthy food choices? Why or why not? Using a food journal to lay it all out can also be extremely helpful.

3. Did you drink at least eight 8-ounce glasses of water each day this week? Ideally, you'll want to aim for more water, especially when exercising, but that would be a solid start!

4. How did you sleep this week? Did you manage to get eight hours of sleep a night? You can work on your sleep hygiene and make tweaks as you go to get a better night's rest.

Notes:

Week Two

"I was always looking outside myself for strength and confidence, but it comes from within. It is there all the time."

—Anna Freud

Welcome to week two! You should be proud of yourself for learning new routines and exercises and developing healthy new habits. Now, it's time to continue down the trail you have blazed.

When you come from a place of nourishing your body and caring for it instead of punishing it, you'll find it much easier to comply with your fitness and health plans. It's all about your viewpoint. To encourage yourself, try repeating an affirmation such as this:

"I enjoy taking care of my body and feeding it nutritious foods. Exercise feels good, and I look forward to it."

WEEK TWO: HOME WORKOUT

Days of the Week: Three nonconsecutive days

Approximate Workout Time: 1 hour, 15 minutes (including a 5-minute warm-up and a 10-minute cool-down)

Overview: Your second week will have you doing a full-body exercise program 3 days a week again. However, in the resistance-training portion, instead of 1 set per body part, you'll increase to 2 sets this week, 12 to 15 repetitions per set.

Reminder: Aim for 60 seconds of rest in between sets and 2 minutes of rest in between body parts.

1 Warm-Up

Start with a gentle 5-minute warm-up. You can walk, jog lightly in place, do some arm circles, climb the stairs; do something endurance-based that gets your heart rate up.

2 Balance Training

1. One-Legged Stand

(page 108) – Hold your leg off the ground for a count of 5, then do 5 repetitions on each side.

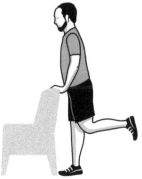

2. Weight Shifts

(page 109) – Do alternating leg lifts until you've done 10 repetitions on each side.

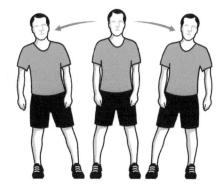

3. Toe Taps

(page 113) – Start slowly and see if you can increase your tapping speed. Go for 15 to 20 seconds.

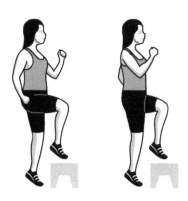

4. Arm Sequence with Lifted Heels

(page 112) – Try to do 20 repetitions in a row.

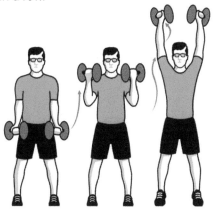

3 Resistance Training

This week, you'll be doing 2 sets of each exercise with 12 to 15 repetitions each time. Make sure the weight feels heavy for you during the last few repetitions on each set. Take 60 seconds between sets and a full 2 minutes of rest between body parts.

1. Dumbbell Chest Press

(page 47)

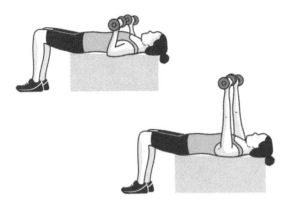

2. Dumbbell Overhead Press

(page 53)

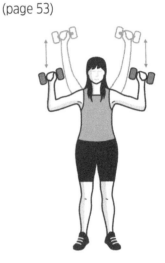

3. Dumbbell Kickback

(page 61) – Do these one arm at a time or with both arms together.

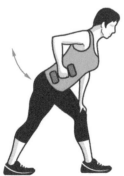

4. Bent-Over Dumbbell Row

(page 65) – Do these one arm at a time or with both arms together.

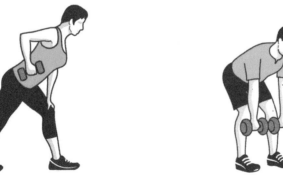
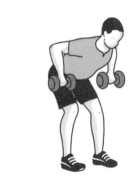

5. Glute Bridge

(page 74)

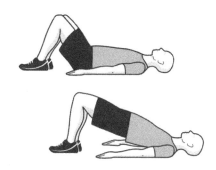

6. Seated Dumbbell Calf Raise

(page 81) – Do 15 to
20 repetitions.

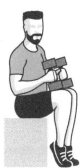

7. Crunch

(page 85) – Do 1 to 2 sets of
20 repetitions.

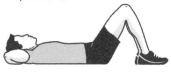

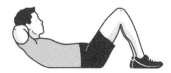

4 Endurance Training

This week, increase your endurance training to 20 minutes. Remember, it should be somewhat challenging, but you shouldn't be completely out of breath. Try to pick up the pace a little this week.

5 Flexibility Training

Finish up and cool down with some flexibility training. Hold each stretch for a count of 10.

1. Quadriceps Stretch
(page 92)

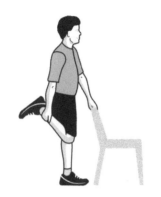

2. Hamstring Stretch
(page 93)

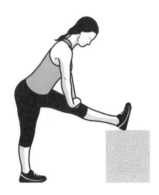

3. Chest Stretch
(page 97)

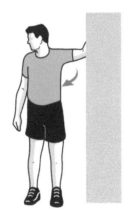

4. Back Stretch
(page 96)

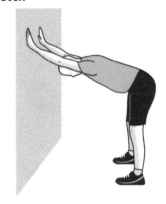

5. Inner-Thigh Stretch
(page 94)

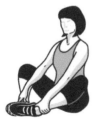

6. Torso Twists
(page 100)

WEEK TWO: GYM WORKOUT

Days of the Week: Three nonconsecutive days

Approximate Workout Time: 1 hour, 15 minutes (including a 5-minute warm-up and a 10-minute cool-down)

Overview: Your second week of workouts will have you doing a full-body exercise program 3 days a week again. However, in the resistance-training portion, instead of 1 set per body part, you'll increase to 2 sets this week, 12 to 15 repetitions per set.

Reminder: Aim for 60 seconds of rest between sets and 2 minutes of rest between body parts.

1 Warm-Up

Start with a gentle 5-minute warm-up. You can walk or jog on the treadmill, use the elliptical trainer, or stair climber.

2 Balance Training

1. One-Legged Stand

(page 108) – Hold your leg off the ground for a count of 5; do 5 repetitions on each side.

2. Weight Shifts

(page 109) – Do alternating leg lifts until you've done 10 repetitions on each side.

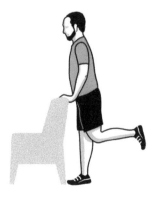

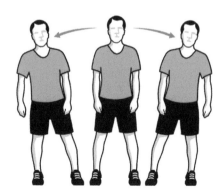

3. Toe Taps

(page 113) – Start slowly and see if you can increase your tapping speed. Go for 15 to 20 seconds.

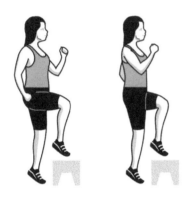

4. Arm Sequence with Lifted Heels

(page 112) – Try to do 20 repetitions in a row.

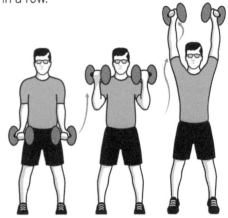

3 Resistance Training

This week, you'll be doing 2 sets of each exercise with 12 to 15 repetitions each time. Make sure the weight feels heavy for you during the last few repetitions of each set. Take 60 seconds between sets and a full 2 minutes of rest between body parts.

1. Dumbbell or Banded Flies

(page 49)

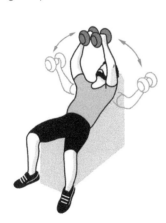

2. Shoulder Press Machine

(page 55)

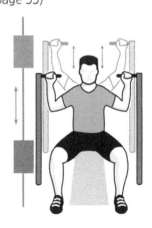

3. Dumbbell Kickback
(page 61)

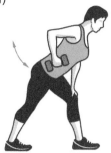

4. Lat Pulldown
(page 69)

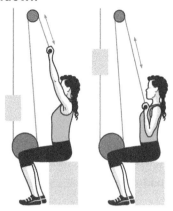

5. Leg Press
(page 79) – Try placing your feet high and wide on the platform to target your glutes.

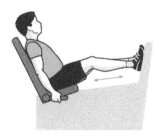

6. Leg Press Calf Raises
(page 83) – Using the Leg Press machine, slide your feet down to the bottom edge of the platform so that just your toes are touching it. Do 15 to 20 repetitions.

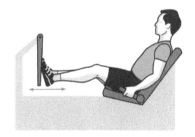

7. Crunch
(page 85) – Do 1 to 2 sets of 20 repetitions.

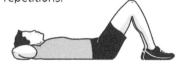

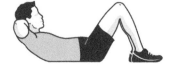

4 Endurance Training

Increase your endurance training to 20 minutes. Try to pick up the pace a little this week.

5 Flexibility Training

Finish up and cool down with some flexibility training. Hold each stretch for a count of 10 and run through the stretches twice.

Quadriceps Stretch
(page 92)

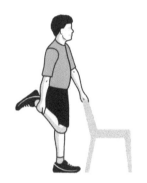

Hamstring Stretch
(page 93)

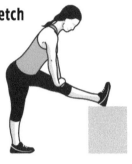

Chest Stretch
(page 97)

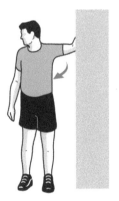

Back Stretch
(page 96)

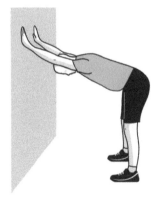

Inner-Thigh Stretch
(page 94)

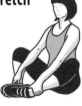

Torso Twists
(page 100)

Week Two: Weekly Check-In

1. How did you feel going through the program this week versus last week? Were you sore? Did you feel a little bit more confident with the movements? Did you feel any stronger? (If not, don't worry; strength takes time!)

2. Did you start a food journal either on paper or online? Did you notice any positive or negative changes in your diet? Were you more or less hungry than usual?

3. Did you get in all the water you needed? If not, try bringing a water bottle with you to your workouts and sipping from it between sets.

4. How was your recovery this week? Did you feel refreshed between workouts or did you need a little extra time to rest? Did you sleep better now that you're exercising more? Have you set up your bedroom for quality sleep?

Notes:

Week Three

"Accept yourself, love yourself, and keep moving forward. If you want to fly, you have to give up what weighs you down."

—Roy T. Bennett

Your body adapts quickly to exercise, and when you plateau it can be tempting to throw in the towel. But this is exactly the time to recommit! Try this affirmation to help you through: "Slower progress is still forward progress. Quitting is not an option, and I will stay the course."

WEEK THREE: HOME WORKOUT

Days of the Week: This week, you will be doing a full-body exercise program for 3 days.

Approximate Workout Time: 1 hour (including a 5-minute warm-up and a 10-minute cool-down)

Overview: This week, start with a 5- to 10-minute warm-up (like walking) and immediately proceed to your resistance training. Take 10 to 15 minutes to cool down with balance-training.

Two days of the week, when you're not doing your resistance-training program, you'll do your endurance and flexibility training. For example, you might lift weights on Monday, Wednesday, and Friday and do endurance exercises on Tuesday and Thursday, with weekends off. Mix it up in a way that works for your schedule.

Reminder: Remember to pick 3 nonconsecutive days to weight train. You want to make sure to have at least 1 day between resistance workouts so that your body has time to recover and you're not doing the same exercises 2 days in a row.

1 Warm-Up

Start with a gentle 5- to 10-minute warm-up. You can walk, do some arm circles, climb the stairs, or jog in place.

2 Resistance Training

Go through these exercises, doing 3 sets of each exercise for 12 to 15 repetitions each, unless otherwise noted. Rest for 60 seconds between repetitions and take 2 minutes of rest between sets.

1. Regular Push-up

(page 46)

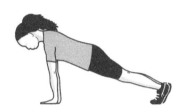

2. Dumbbell Hammer Curls

(page 57)

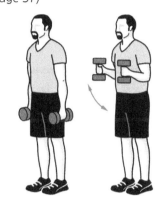

3. Banded Seated Row

(page 66)

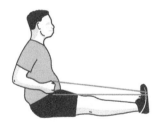

4. Walking Lunge

(page 76)

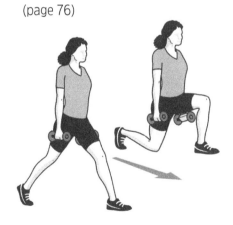

5. Stability Ball Hamstring Roll-In
(page 77)

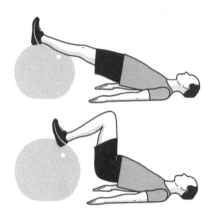

6. Standing Banded Calf Raise
(page 82) – Do 15 to 20 repetitions.

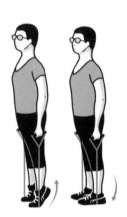

3 Endurance Training

This week, because your endurance-training sessions are getting longer, you'll split up your resistance-training days and your endurance-training days. On the days you do endurance training, go for 30 to 40 minutes.

4 Balance Training

You'll be doing 10 to 15 minutes of balance training after your weight training as part of your cool-down. Do 15 to 20 repetitions of each exercise and go through the entire sequence twice if time allows.

1. Weight Shifts
(page 109)

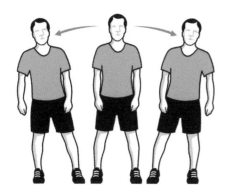

2. Standing Crunch with Under-Leg Clap
(page 110)

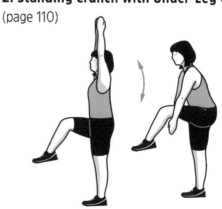

3. Arm Sequence with Lifted Heels
(page 112)

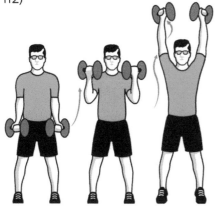

4. Tightrope Walk
(page 106)

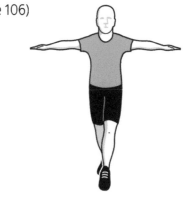

5. Side Leg Raise
(page 107)

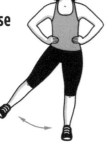

5 Flexibility Training

Finish up and cool down after your endurance training with some flexibility training. Hold each stretch for a count of 10. Run through the exercises 3 times each.

1. Quadriceps Stretch

(page 92)

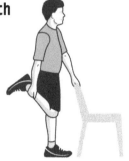

2. Chest Stretch

(page 97)

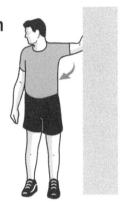

3. Back Stretch

(page 96)

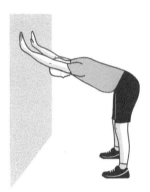

4. Hip Stretch

(page 98)

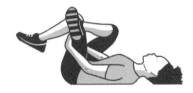

5. Overhead Triceps Stretch

(page 99)

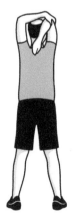

WEEK THREE: GYM WORKOUT

Days of the Week: This week, you will be doing a full-body exercise program for 3 days.

Approximate Workout Time: 1 hour (including a 5-minute warm-up and a 10-minute cool-down)

Overview: This week, you'll start with a 5- to 10-minute warm-up and immediately proceed to your resistance training. After your resistance training, you'll take 10 to 15 minutes to cool down with the balance-training exercises.

Two days of the week, when you're not doing your resistance-training program, you'll do your endurance and flexibility training. For example, you might lift weights on Monday, Wednesday, and Friday and do endurance exercises on Tuesday and Thursday, with weekends off.

Reminder: Make sure to have at least 1 day between resistance workouts so that your body has time to recover and you're not doing the same exercises 2 days in a row.

1 Warm-Up

Start with a gentle 5- to 10-minute warm-up like a gentle treadmill jog or slow pedaling on a bike.

2 Resistance Training

Go through these exercises, doing 3 sets of each exercise for 12 to 15 repetitions each, unless otherwise noted. Rest for 60 seconds between repetitions and take 2 minutes of rest between sets.

1. Lateral Shoulder Raise Machine
(page 56)

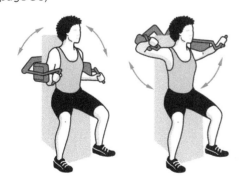

2. Dumbbell Hammer Curls
(page 57)

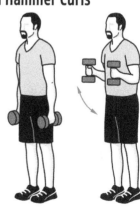

3. Seated Cable Row
(page 70)

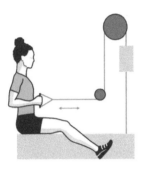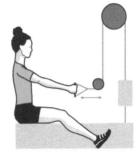

4. Dumbbell Squat
(page 75)

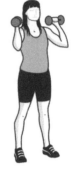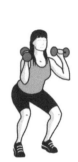

5. Hamstring Curl
(page 80)

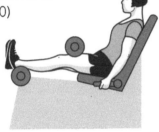

6. Standing Banded Calf Raise
(page 82) – Do 15 to 20 repetitions.

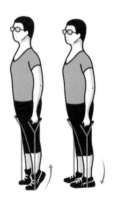

7. Hanging Leg Raises
(page 87)

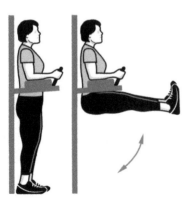

3 Endurance Training

This week, because your endurance-training sessions are getting longer, you'll split up your resistance-training days and your endurance-training days. On the days you do endurance training, go for 30 to 40 minutes.

4 Balance Training

You'll be doing 10 to 15 minutes of balance training as part of your cool-down. Do 15 to 20 repetitions of each exercise and repeat the entire sequence twice.

1. Weight Shifts
(page 109)

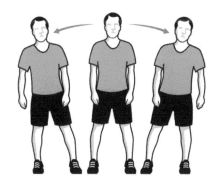

2. Standing Crunch with Under-Leg Clap
(page 110)

3. Arm Sequence with Lifted Heels
(page 112)

4. Tightrope Walk
(page 106)

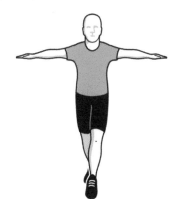

5. Side Leg Raise

(page 107)

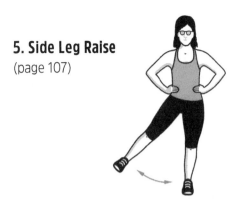

5 Flexibility Training

Finish up and cool down after your endurance training with some flexibility training. Hold each stretch for a count of 10. Repeat the exercises 3 times each.

1. Quadriceps Stretch

(page 92)

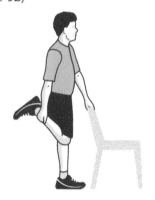

2. Chest Stretch

(page 97)

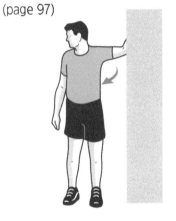

3. Back Stretch

(page 96)

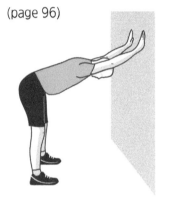

4. Hip Stretch

(page 98)

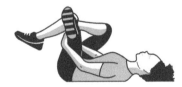

5. Overhead Triceps Stretch

(page 99)

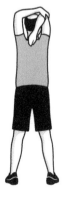

Week Three: Weekly Check-In

Your week-three check-in will help make sure you are feeling good about your program and you are staying on track. You should be monitoring your progress every week and starting to see some real changes in your body and your health.

1. Are you feeling more energized now that you're eating healthy, whole, nutritious foods? If you're viewing your meals as fuel for your workouts, is this strategy helping you?

2. Are you continuing to get enough water each day? Beyond the water bottle, improve your hydration by eating foods with a high water content, such as fruits, melons, and fibrous vegetables.

3. Did you find yourself recovering well this week? Did you have enough energy for your workouts, thanks to your food choices and hydration?

4. How is the workout plan going? Are you enjoying the exercise selection? Are you continuing to monitor your progress?

Notes:

Week Four

"Discipline is built by consistently performing small acts of courage."

—Robin Sharma

You've built healthy habits, and the longer you practice them, the more natural they will become. If you find yourself struggling this week, try repeating an affirmation such as this:

"I am grateful that I get to exercise and eat in a healthy way. My positive outlook is contagious, my mindset is strength, and my attitude is happiness. I choose happy and fit."

WEEK FOUR: HOME WORKOUT

Days of the Week: This week, you will be doing 3 days of a full-body exercise program and 2 days of endurance training.

Approximate Workout Time: 1 hour, 15 minutes (including a 5-minute warm-up and a 15-minute cool-down)

Overview: On your 3 days of resistance training, start with a 5- to 10-minute warm-up (like walking). Do 3 sets of each exercise, aiming to go a little heavier than last week. Cut your rest time down to 90 seconds. After weight training, round out with 15 minutes of balance exercises.

On non-resistance-training days, do 45 minutes of endurance training followed by 15 minutes of flexibility training. For example, if you do resistance on Monday, Wednesday, and Friday, you'll do endurance on Tuesday and Thursday or a weekend day.

Reminder: Make sure to have at least 1 day between resistance workouts so that your body has time to recover and you're not doing the same exercises 2 days in a row.

1 Warm-Up

For 5 minutes, walk or run up and down the stairs a few times, jog in place, or do something else that will get your heart rate up.

2 Resistance Training

You are now up to 3 sets of each exercise, with 12 to 15 repetitions for each. Take 60 seconds of rest between sets and 90 seconds of rest between body parts.

1. Regular Push-Ups

(page 46)

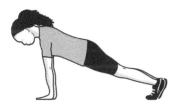

2. Lying Banded Chest Press

(page 48)

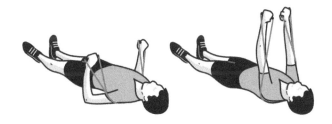

3. Dumbbell Lateral Shoulder Raise

(page 52)

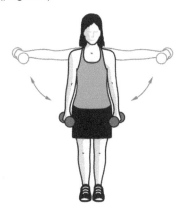

4. Banded Overhead Shoulder Press

(page 54)

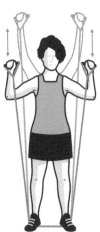

5. Dumbbell Hammer Curls
(page 57)

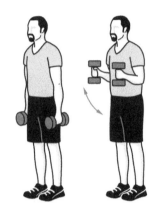

6. Standing Banded Biceps Curl
(page 58)

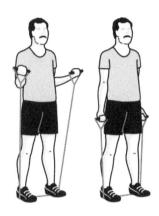

7. Triceps Dip
(page 60)

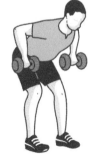

8. Superman
(page 64)

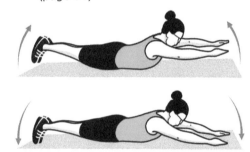

9. Bent-Over Dumbbell Row
(page 65)

10. Dumbbell Squat
(page 75)

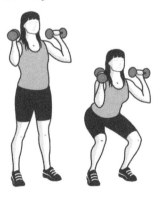

11. Standing Banded Calf Raise
(page 82)

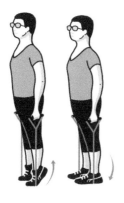

12. Plank
(page 84)

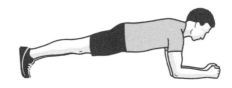

13. Crunch
(page 85)

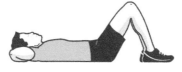
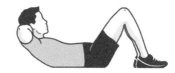

3 Endurance Training

Two days per week, when you're not weight training, do 45 minutes of endurance training. Try 15 minutes of walking, 15 minutes of jogging, and a 15-minute bike ride.

4 Balance Training

You'll be doing 10 to 15 minutes of balance training on your weight-training days as part of your cool-down. Do 15 to 20 repetitions of each exercise and repeat the entire sequence twice.

1. Weight Shifts
(page 109)

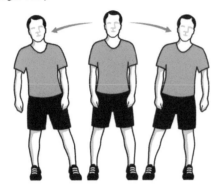

2. Toe Taps
(page 113)

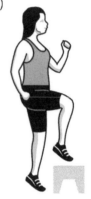 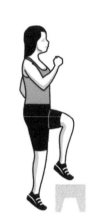

3. Standing Crunch with Under-Leg Clap
(page 110)

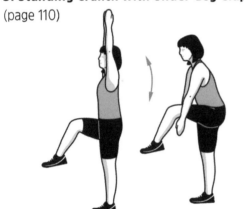

4. Rolling Forearm Side Plank
(page 111)

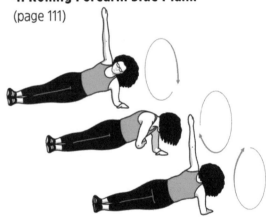

5. Tightrope Walk
(page 106)

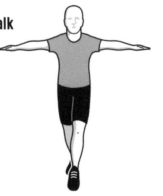

6. Side Leg Raise
(page 107)

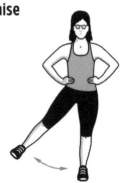

5 Flexibility Training

On endurance days, cool down with 15 minutes of flexibility training. Hold each stretch for a count of 10. Repeat all flexibility exercises 3 times.

1. Quadriceps Stretch
(page 92)

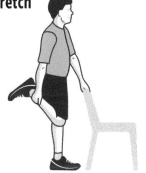

2. Hamstring Stretch
(page 93)

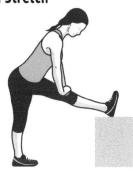

3. Inner-Thigh Stretch
(page 94)

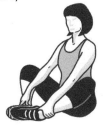

4. Calf Stretch
(page 95)

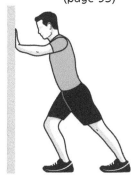
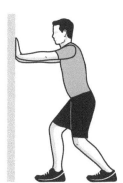

5. Back Stretch
(page 96)

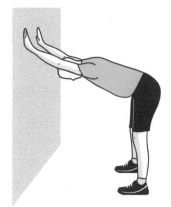

6. Chest Stretch
(page 97)

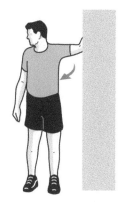

7. Hip Stretch
(page 98)

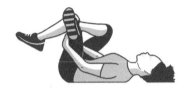

8. Overhead Triceps Stretch
(page 99)

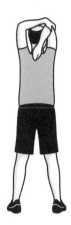

WEEK FOUR: GYM WORKOUT

Days of the Week: This week, you will be doing 3 days of a full body exercise program and 2 days of endurance training.

Approximate Workout Time: 1 hour, 15 minutes (including a 5-minute warm-up and a 10-minute cool-down)

Overview: On your 3 days of resistance training, start with a 5- to 10-minute warm-up (something like walking). Then you'll do 3 sets for each exercise but try to go a little heavier than you did last week and reduce your rest time between body parts down to 90 seconds. After your weight training, you'll round out the session with about 15 minutes of balance exercises.

On the days you're not doing resistance training, you'll do 45 minutes of endurance training followed by 15 minutes of flexibility training. Aim for 2 days of endurance training this week. For example, if you do resistance training on Monday, Wednesday, and Friday, you'll do endurance training on Tuesday and Thursday or a weekend day.

Reminder: Remember to pick 3 nonconsecutive days to weight train. You want to make sure to have at least 1 day between resistance workouts so that your body has time to recover and you're not doing the same exercises 2 days in a row.

1 Warm-Up

Start with a gentle 5-minute warm-up. You can walk on a treadmill with a slight incline, ride a recumbent bike, or jump rope—whatever gets your heart rate up.

2 Resistance Training

You are now up to 3 sets of 12 to 15 repetitions for each exercise. Take 60 seconds of rest between sets and 90 seconds of rest between body parts.

1. Regular Push-Ups

(page 46)

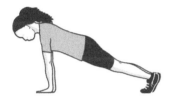

2. Pec Dec Chest Fly Machine

(page 51)

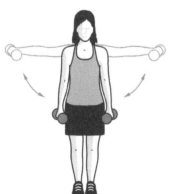

3. Dumbbell Lateral Shoulder Raise

(page 52)

4. Shoulder Press Machine

(page 55)

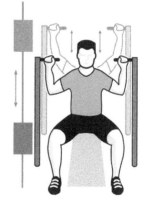

5. Dumbbell Hammer Curls
(page 57)

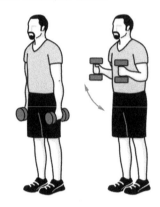

6. Standing Banded Biceps Curl
(page 58)

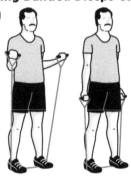

7. Triceps Cable Pushdown
(page 63)

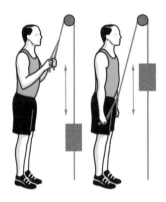

8. Lat Pulldown
(page 69)

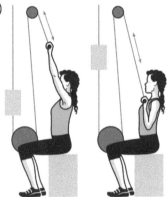

9. Seated Cable Row
(page 70)

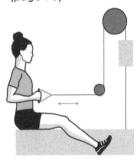
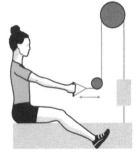

10. Dumbbell Romanian Deadlift
(page 78)

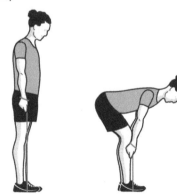

11. Leg Press
(page 79)

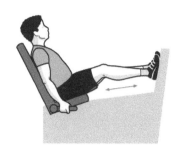

12. Seated Dumbbell Calf Raise
(page 81)

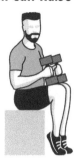

13. Stability Ball Knee-Ins
(page 86)

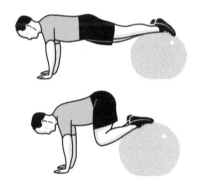

14. Hanging Leg Raises
(page 87)

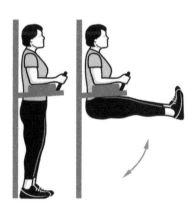

3 Endurance Training

Two days per week, when you're not weight training, you'll be doing 45 minutes of endurance training. Try 15 minutes on the stepper or stair climber followed by 15 minutes on a bike. Finish it off with a light 15-minute treadmill jog.

4 Balance Training

You'll be doing 10 to 15 minutes of balance training after your weight training as part of your cool-down. Do 15 to 20 repetitions of each exercise and repeat the entire sequence twice.

1. Weight Shifts
(page 109)

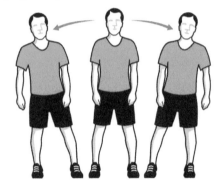

2. Toe Taps
(page 113)

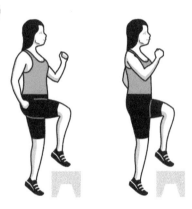

3. Standing Crunch with Under-Leg Clap
(page 110)

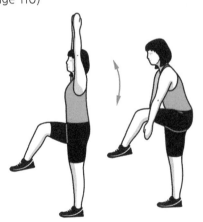

4. Rolling Forearm Side Plank
(page 111)

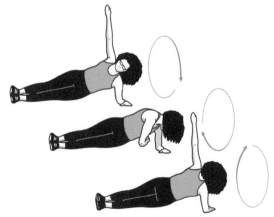

5. Tightrope Walk
(page 106)

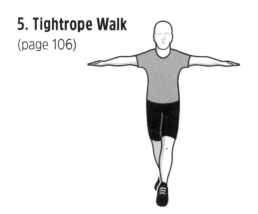

6. Side Leg Raise
(page 107)

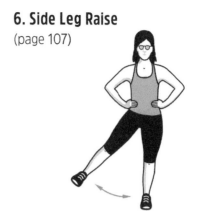

5 Flexibility Training

Cool down with 15 minutes of flexibility training. Hold each stretch for a count of 10. Repeat all flexibility exercises 3 times.

1. Quadriceps Stretch
(page 92)

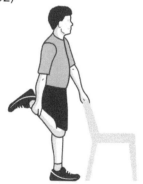

2. Hamstring Stretch
(page 93)

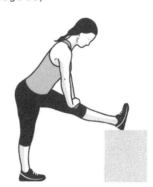

3. Inner-Thigh Stretch
(page 94)

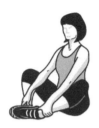

4. Calf Stretch
(page 95)

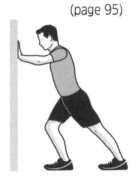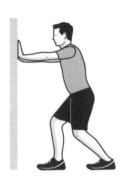

5. Back Stretch
(page 96)

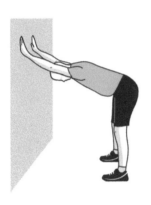

6. Chest Stretch
(page 97)

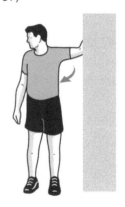

7. Hip Stretch
(page 98)

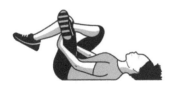

8. Overhead Triceps Stretch
(page 99)

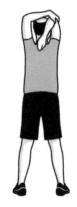

Week Four: Weekly Check-In

Now that you've made it this far, it's time for a reward! It's important to have goals to keep you focused and moving forward, but rewarding yourself for reaching those goals is also key!

1. How are you feeling at this point? Take some time to reflect upon how far you've come. How will you reward yourself? What types of non-food rewards can you look forward to in the future?

2. Has your nutrition been on point this week? Why or why not? You may find it more manageable to eat healthy six days a week and then look forward to one "cheat meal" of your choice on a weekly basis.

3. Has your exercise and sleep schedule become routine? Or do you find you're still struggling to make time for exercise and to get to bed on time? Making yourself a priority and reviewing your goals and your "whys" and can help you get on track.

4. Are you finding the improvements you've made to be motivating and exciting? Do you want to learn more about your fitness and health? Remember, it's okay to take care of yourself. Besides, if you're healthy and fit, you'll be in a much better place to help others.

Notes:

Week Five

"The key is not to prioritize your schedule, but to schedule your priorities."

—Stephen Covey

Welcome to week five. Now, your fitness should start feeling like a normal part of your routine. This is how healthy habits are made! This week, try repeating an affirmation such as this:

"I live a fitness lifestyle, and it is simply a part of who I am."

WEEK FIVE: HOME WORKOUT

Days of the Week: This week, you will be working your upper body and your lower body separately.

Approximate Workout Time: 1 hour

Overview: Your fifth week will have you splitting the body into upper and lower parts. You'll do 2 days of upper-body workouts and 2 days of lower-body workouts, along with 2 days of endurance training, for a 6-day workout week.

Here's an example of what it could look like:

Monday—upper-body and balance training

Tuesday—lower-body and balance training

Wednesday—endurance and flexibility training

Thursday—upper-body and balance training

Friday—lower-body and balance training

Saturday—endurance and flexibility training

Sunday—OFF

Reminder: If you don't want to work out this often, do an upper-body training day followed by an endurance-training day, followed by a lower-body training day. You can also spread the program out and take rest days in between.

1 Warm-Up

Start with a gentle 5- to 10-minute warm-up. Then, for this week's resistance training days, do 1 set of each exercise for 12 to 15 repetitions. Rest for 60 seconds between sets and 90 seconds between body parts.

2 Resistance Training – Upper Body

1. Dumbbell Chest Press
(page 47)

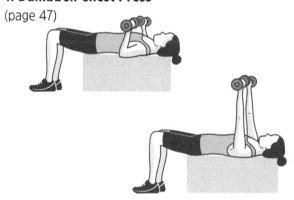

2. Dumbbell or Banded Flies
(page 49)

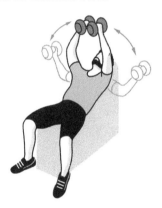

3. Dumbbell Lateral Shoulder Raise
(page 52)

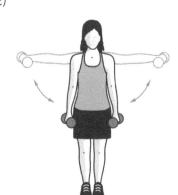

4. Dumbbell Overhead Press
(page 53)

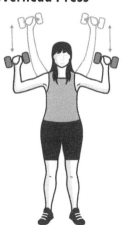

5. Dumbbell Hammer Curls
(page 57)

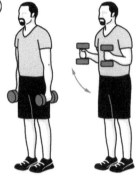

6. Triceps Dip
(page 60)

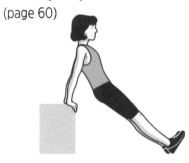

7. Dumbbell Kickback
(page 61)

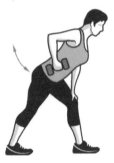

8. Bent-Over Dumbbell Row
(page 65)

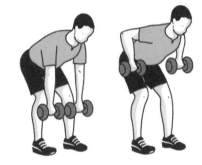

9. Banded Seated Row
(page 66)

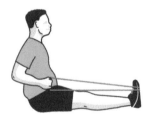

3 Resistance Training – Lower Body

1. Squat
(page 73)

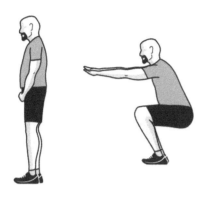

2. Glute Bridge
(page 74)

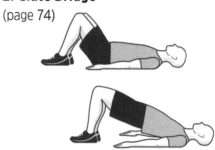

3. Walking Lunge
(page 76)

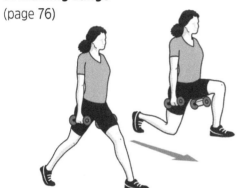

4. Stability Ball Hamstring Roll-In
(page 77)

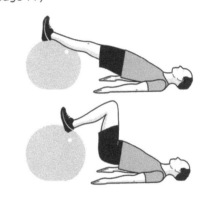

5. Banded Romanian Deadlift
(page 78)

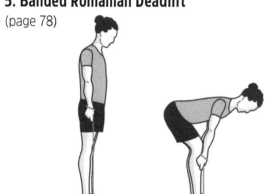

6. Seated Dumbbell Calf Raise
(page 81)

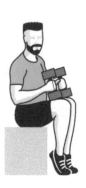

7. Standing Banded Calf Raise
(page 82)

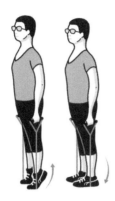

4 Balance Training

You'll be doing 10 to 15 minutes of balance training after your resistance training. Do 15 to 20 repetitions of each exercise and go through the entire sequence twice if time allows.

1. Weight Shifts
(page 109)

2. Toe Taps
(page 113)

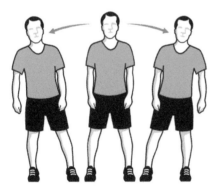

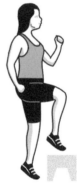
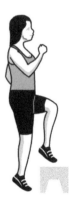

3. Standing Crunch with Under-Leg Clap
(page 110)

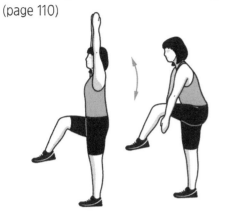

4. Rolling Forearm Side Plank
(page 111)

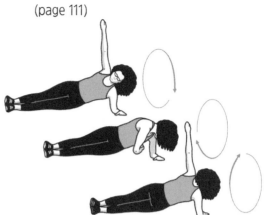

5. Tightrope Walk
(page 106)

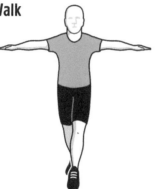

6. Side Leg Raise
(page 107)

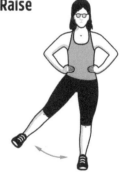

7. One-Legged Stand
(page 108)

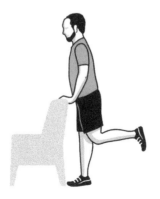

8. Arm Sequence with Lifted Heels
(page 112)

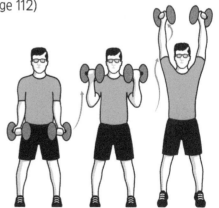

5 Flexibility Training

Cool down after your endurance training with 15 minutes of flexibility training. Hold each stretch for a count of 10. Repeat all flexibility exercises 3 times.

1. Overhead Triceps Stretch

(page 99)

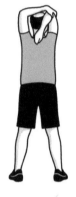

2. Hip Stretch

(page 98)

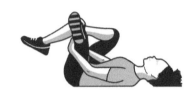

3. Chest Stretch

(page 97)

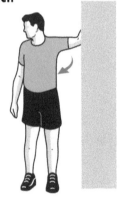

4. Arm Circles

(page 99)

5. Cat Cow

(page 100)

6. Torso Twists

(page 100)

7. Leg Pendulums

(page 100)

WEEK FIVE: GYM WORKOUT

Days of the Week: This week, you will be working your upper body and your lower body separately.

Approximate Workout Time: 1 hour

Overview: Your fifth week will have you splitting the body into upper and lower parts. You'll do 2 days of upper-body workouts and 2 days of lower-body workouts, along with 2 days of endurance training, for a 6-day workout week. Revisit page 160 for a suggested schedule.

Reminder: If you don't want to work out this often, you can simply do an upper-body training day followed by an endurance-training day, followed by a lower-body training day. You can also spread the program out and take rest days in between.

1 Warm-Up

Start with a gentle 5- to 10-minute warm-up. Just get the blood moving before you begin your weight training. You'll do 1 set of each exercise for 12 to 15 repetitions. Rest for 60 seconds between sets and 90 seconds between body parts.

2 Resistance Training – Upper Body

1. Seated Chest Press
(page 50)

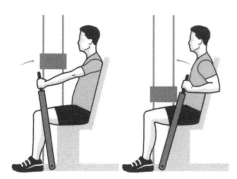

2. Pec Dec Chest Fly Machine
(page 51)

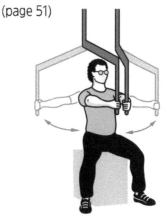

3. Lateral Shoulder Raise Machine
(page 56)

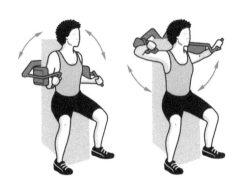

4. Dumbbell Overhead Press
(page 53)

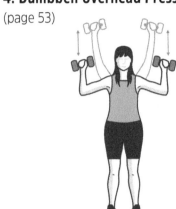

5. Preacher Curl
(page 59)

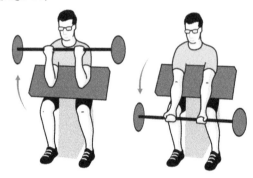

6. Dumbbell Hammer Curls
(page 57)

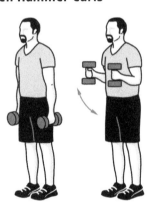

7. Triceps Cable Pushdown
(page 63)

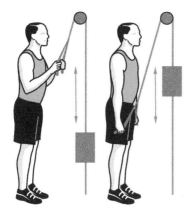

8. Dumbbell Kickback
(page 61)

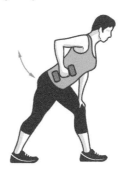

9. Seated Cable Row
(page 70)

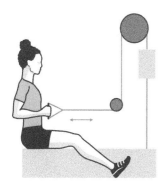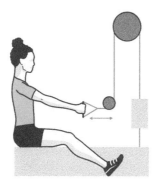

10. Pull-Ups or Assisted Pull-Ups
(page 71)

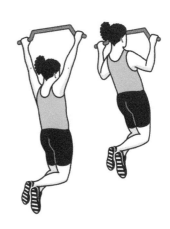

3 Resistance Training – Lower Body

1. Leg Press
(page 79)

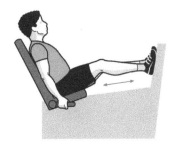

2. Glute Bridge
(page 74)

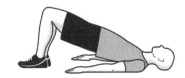

3. Walking Lunge
(page 76)

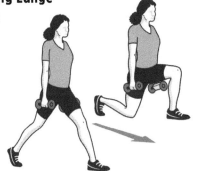

4. Hamstring Curl
(page 80)

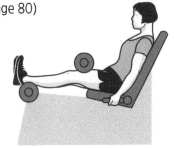

5. Dumbbell Romanian Deadlift
(page 78)

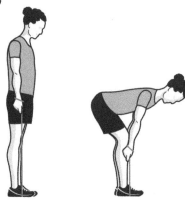

6. Seated Dumbbell Calf Raise
(page 81)

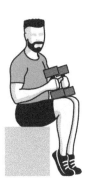

7. Leg Press Calf Raises
(page 83)

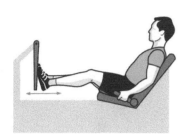

8. Stability Ball Knee-Ins
(page 86)

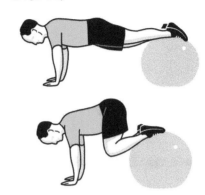

9. Hanging Leg Raises
(page 87)

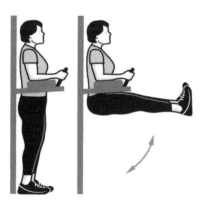

4 Balance Training

You'll be doing 10 to 15 minutes of balance training after your weight training as part of your cool-down. Do 15 to 20 repetitions of each exercise and repeat the entire sequence twice.

1. Weight Shifts
(page 109)

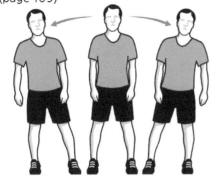

2. Toe Taps
(page 113)

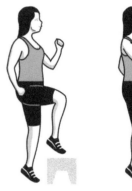
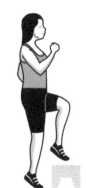

3. Standing Crunch with Under-Leg Clap
(page 110)

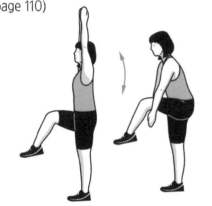

4. Rolling Forearm Side Plank
(page 111)

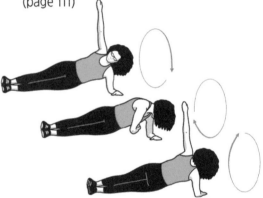

5. Tightrope Walk
(page 106)

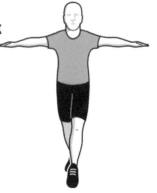
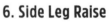

6. Side Leg Raise
(page 107)

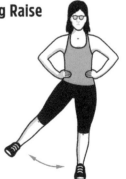

7. One-Legged Stand
(page 108)

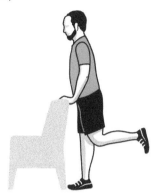

8. Arm Sequence with Lifted Heels
(page 112)

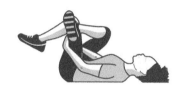

5 Flexibility Training

Finish up and cool down after your endurance training with 15 minutes of flexibility training. Hold each stretch for a count of 10. Repeat all flexibility exercises 3 times.

1. Overhead Triceps Stretch
(page 99)

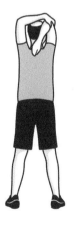

2. Hip Stretch
(page 98)

3. Chest Stretch
(page 97)

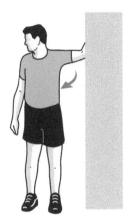

4. Arm Circles
(page 99)

5. Cat Cow
(page 100)

6. Torso Twists
(page 100)

7. Leg Pendulums
(page 100)

Week Five: Weekly Check-In

Great job working out this week and getting to week five of your program! You should be extremely proud of yourself.

1. How are you feeling? Is your body feeling stronger? If at any point, you feel like you're not progressing, simply repeat the last week of workouts until you're ready to move forward.

2. Have your nutrition and hydration been on point this week? Are you feeling better about your fitness now that positive actions are becoming part of your routine?

3. Have other people started to notice your success and the positive changes you've made? Are you noticing motivating changes both in the mirror and within yourself?

Notes:

Week Six

> "You are the leader you've been looking for."
>
> —Maria Shriver

Now that you are entering week six of your workout program, you should be excited by your progress. This is what you're all about: setting and achieving goals. This week, try repeating an affirmation such as this:

"When I have a goal in mind, I make plans and I take action to achieve it."

WEEK SIX: HOME WORKOUT

Days of the Week: This week, you will be working your upper body and your lower body separately.

Approximate Workout Time: 1 hour

Overview: This week, you will again be splitting the body into upper and lower body parts. You'll do 2 days of upper-body workouts and 2 days of lower-body workouts, along with 2 days of endurance training, for a 6-day workout week. Revisit page 160 for a suggested schedule.

Reminder: If these workouts have progressed too quickly, simply go back to the weeks that worked best for you and repeat those until you're comfortable moving forward. Or, simply add additional rest days into the program between training days.

1 Warm-Up

Start with a gentle 5- to 10-minute warm-up. You can walk, jog lightly in place, do some arm circles, or climb the stairs—whatever gets your heart rate up. You'll do 2 sets of each exercise for 12 to 15 repetitions. Rest for 60 seconds between sets and 90 seconds between body parts.

2 Resistance Training – Upper Body

1. Dumbbell Chest Press
(page 47)

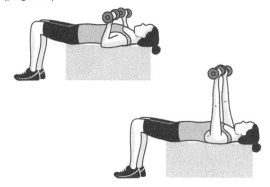

2. Dumbbell or Banded Flies
(page 49)

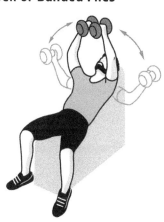

3. Dumbbell Lateral Shoulder Raise
(page 52)

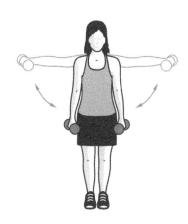

4. Dumbbell Overhead Press
(page 53)

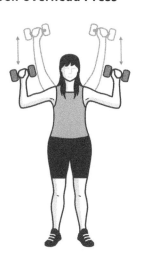

5. Dumbbell Hammer Curls

(page 57)

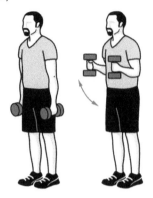

6. Triceps Dip

(page 60)

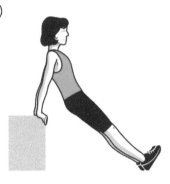

7. Dumbbell Kickback

(page 61)

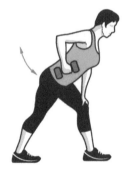

8. Bent-Over Dumbbell Row

(page 65)

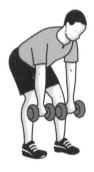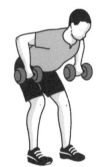

9. Banded Seated Row

(page 66)

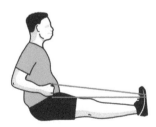

3 Resistance Training – Lower Body

1. Squat
(page 73)

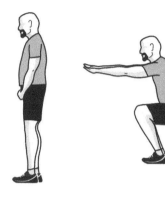

2. Glute Bridge
(page 74)

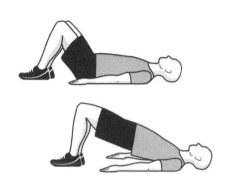

3. Walking Lunge
(page 76)

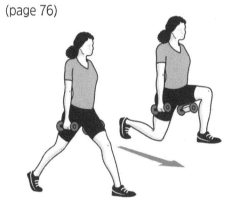

4. Stability Ball Hamstring Roll-In
(page 77)

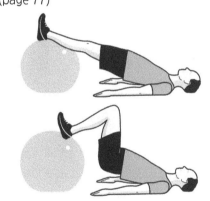

5. Banded Romanian Deadlift
(page 78)

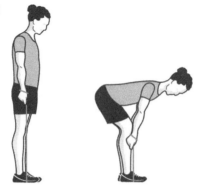

6. Seated Dumbbell Calf Raise
(page 81)

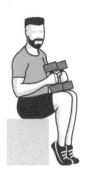

7. Standing Banded Calf Raise
(page 82)

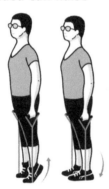

4 Endurance Training

This week, you'll do 10 minutes of high-intensity interval training (HIIT). After your warm-up, you'll do intervals of 15 seconds of maximum effort followed by 45 seconds of "rest," which is continuing to move slowly at a lower level of effort. You'll do 10 rounds of this, and then finish off your regular endurance training for 20 to 30 minutes.

Your HIIT routine might look something like this:

15 seconds fast pedaling on an indoor bike

45 seconds of slower pedaling

Repeat this sequence for 10 rounds

Continue with your favorite form of endurance training for the remaining 20 or 30 minutes, depending on your fitness level.

Note: HIIT isn't for everyone, and not everyone may be ready to commit to it. It's a great way to improve your cardiovascular fitness, but stick with your usual endurance-training routine from the earlier weeks if you feel more comfortable.

5 Balance Training

On days you don't do endurance training, you'll be doing 10 to 15 minutes of balance training after your weight training as part of your cool-down. Do 15 to 20 repetitions of each exercise and repeat the entire sequence twice.

1. Weight Shifts
(page 109)

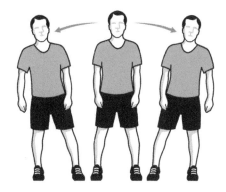

2. Toe Taps
(page 113)

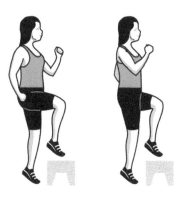

3. Standing Crunch with Under-Leg Clap
(page 110)

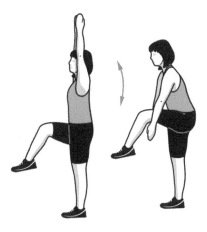

4. Rolling Forearm Side Plank
(page 111)

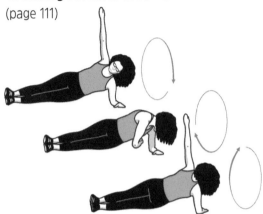

5. Tightrope Walk
(page 106)

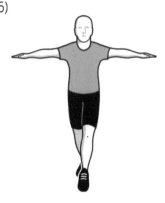

6. Side Leg Raise
(page 107)

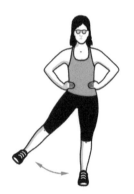

7. One-Legged Stand
(page 108)

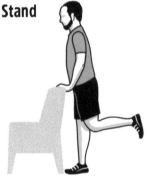

8. Arm Sequence with Lifted Heels
(page 112)

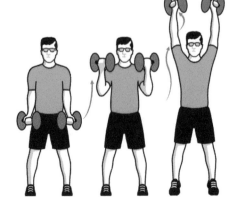

6 Flexibility Training

Cool down after your endurance training with 15 minutes of flexibility training. Hold each stretch for a count of 10. Repeat all flexibility exercises 3 times.

1. Quadriceps Stretch
(page 92)

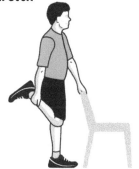

2. Hamstring Stretch
(page 93)

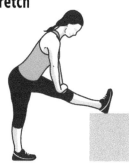

4. Calf Stretch
(page 95)

3. Inner-Thigh Stretch
(page 94)

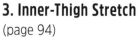
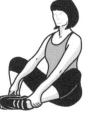
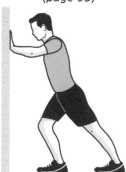
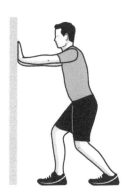

5. Back Stretch
(page 96)

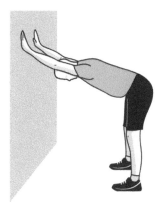

6. Overhead Triceps Stretch
(page 99)

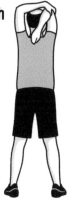

7. Hip Stretch
(page 98)

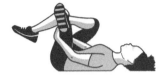

8. Chest Stretch
(page 97)

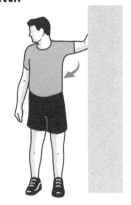

9. Arm Circles
(page 99)

10. Cat Cow
(page 100)

11. Torso Twists
(page 100)

12. Leg Pendulums
(page 100)

WEEK SIX: GYM WORKOUT

Days of the Week: This week, you will be working your upper and your lower body separately.

Approximate Workout Time: 1 hour

Overview: This week, you will again be splitting the body into upper and lower body parts. You'll do 2 days of upper-body workouts and 2 days of lower-body workouts, along with 2 days of endurance training, for a 6-day workout week. Revisit page 160 for a suggested schedule.

Reminder: If you feel like these workouts have progressed too quickly, go back to the weeks that worked best for you and repeat those until you're comfortable with moving forward. Or simply add additional rest days into the program between training days.

1 Warm-Up

Start with a gentle 5- to 10-minute warm-up. You can walk on the treadmill, climb stairs on the stepper, or do some gentle gliding on the elliptical. You'll do 2 sets of each exercise for 12 to 15 repetitions. Rest for 60 seconds between sets and 90 seconds between body parts.

2 Resistance Training – Upper Body

1. Seated Chest Press
(page 50)

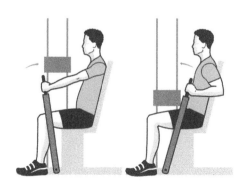

2. Pec Dec Chest Fly Machine
(page 51)

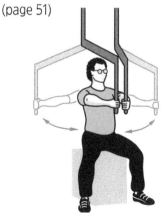

3. Lateral Shoulder Raise Machine
(page 56)

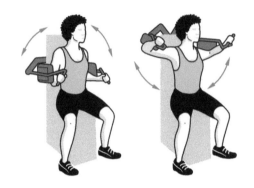

4. Dumbbell Overhead Press
(page 53)

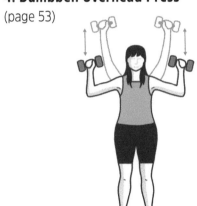

5. Preacher Curl
(page 59)

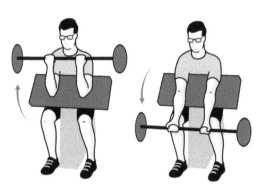

6. Dumbbell Hammer Curls
(page 57)

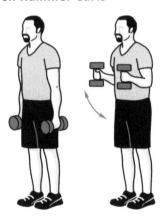

7. Triceps Cable Pushdown
(page 63)

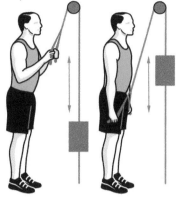

8. Dumbbell Kickback
(page 61)

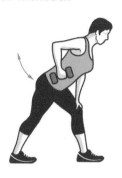

9. Seated Cable Row
(page 70)

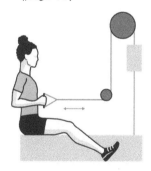
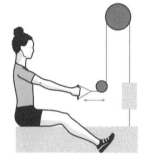

10. Pull-Ups or Assisted Pull-Ups
(page 71)

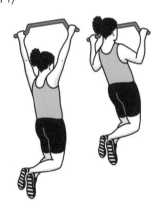

3 Resistance Training – Lower Body

1. Leg Press
(page 79)

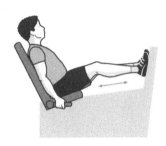

2. Glute Bridge
(page 74)

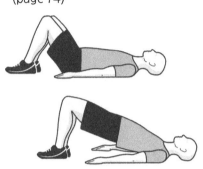

3. Walking Lunge
(page 76)

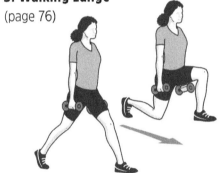

4. Hamstring Curl
(page 80)

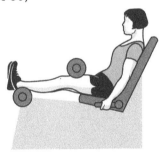

5. Dumbbell Romanian Deadlift
(page 78)

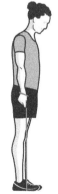
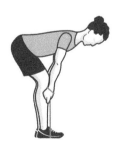

6. Seated Dumbbell Calf Raise
(page 81)

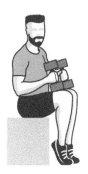

7. Leg Press Calf Raise
(page 83)

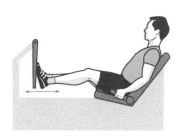

8. Stability Ball Knee-Ins
(page 86)

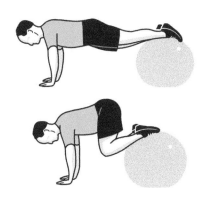

9. Hanging Leg Raises
(page 87)

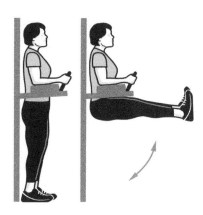

4 Endurance Training

This week, you'll do 10 minutes of high-intensity interval training (HIIT). After your warm-up, you'll do intervals of 15 seconds of maximum effort followed by 45 seconds of "rest," which is continuing to move slowly at a lower level of effort. You'll do 10 rounds of this, and then finish off with your regular endurance training for 20 to 30 minutes.

Your HIIT routine might look something like this:

15 seconds fast pedaling on an indoor bike

45 seconds of slower pedaling

Repeat this sequence for 10 rounds

Continue with your favorite form of endurance training for the remaining 20 or 30 minutes, depending on your fitness level.

Note: HIIT isn't for everyone, and not everyone may be ready to commit to it. It's a great way to improve your cardiovascular fitness, but stick with your usual endurance-training routine from the earlier weeks if you feel more comfortable.

5 Balance Training

On days you don't do endurance training, you'll be doing 10 to 15 minutes of balance training after your weight training as part of your cool-down. Do 15 to 20 repetitions of each exercise and repeat the entire sequence twice.

1. Weight Shifts
(page 109)

2. Toe Taps
(page 113)

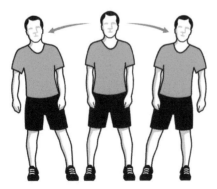 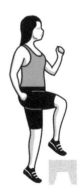 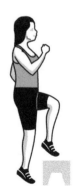

3. Standing Crunch with Under-Leg Clap
(page 110)

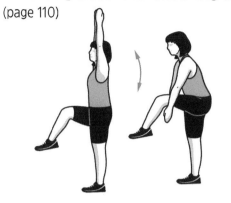

4. Rolling Forearm Side Plank
(page 111)

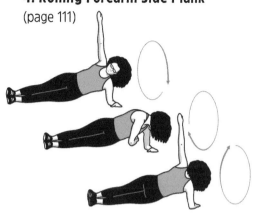

5. Tightrope Walk
(page 106)

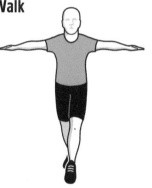

6. Side Leg Raise
(page 107)

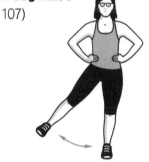

8. Arm Sequence with Lifted Heels
(page 112)

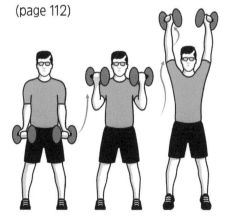

7. One-Legged Stand
(page 108)

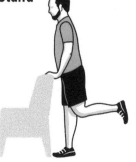

6 Flexibility Training

Finish up and cool down after your endurance training with 15 minutes of flexibility training. Hold each stretch for a count of 10. Repeat all flexibility exercises 3 times.

1. Quadriceps Stretch

(page 92)

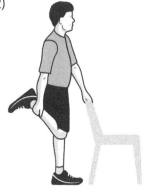

2. Hamstring Stretch

(page 93)

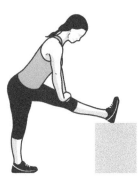

4. Calf Stretch

(page 95)

3. Inner-Thigh Stretch

(page 94)

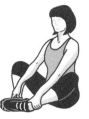

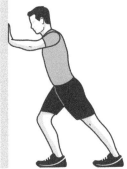

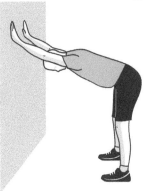

5. Back Stretch

(page 96)

6. Overhead Triceps Stretch
(page 99)

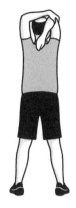

7. Hip Stretch
(page 98)

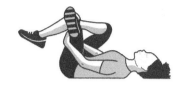

8. Chest Stretch
(page 97)

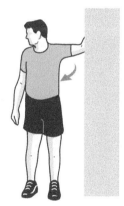

9. Arm Circles
(page 99)

10. Cat Cow
(page 100)

11. Torso Twists
(page 100)

12. Leg Pendulums
(page 100)

Week Six: Weekly Check-In

You did it! You made it to the finish line of your program. You should be extremely proud of yourself. You set a goal, took action, and now you are here.

1. What have you learned about yourself, your health and fitness, and your lifestyle?

2. What did you do well over the past six weeks, and what are some areas for improvement?

3. What will you do to stay motivated as you face challenges moving forward? Have you found social support in friends, family, or online groups?

4. What will you do next to keep up your progress? What are your next fitness goals?

Notes:

9
KEEP IT UP

In this final chapter, we're going to discuss how to keep your forward momentum going and how to head off potential challenges. Life happens, but that doesn't mean you need to get derailed. Keep in mind this isn't about being perfect; it's about being consistent and making your fitness and health priorities in your life.

You Got This!

Success begets success, and the more you keep up with your new fitness lifestyle, the better you'll feel. Your conditioning will improve, and your body will become even stronger. You may even find that your mind is clearer, your energy levels are higher, your sleep improves, and your attitude about life in general is more buoyant.

Once you've completed your six-week program, feel free to mix it up, pick and choose your favorite exercises, add some of your own, or branch out into other areas of fitness. Remember, you can always go back to these same exercises and ramp up the difficulty by increasing the weight and number of repetitions, and decreasing the rest times. Keep challenging yourself!

How Do I Tune In to Myself?

Tuning in to and taking good care of yourself are important facets of a fitness lifestyle. It's important that you continue to get regular medical checkups and monitor your overall health, and that you continue to monitor your physical fitness progress as well. Consider keeping a log of your weight and your measurements. You may want to weigh and measure yourself once a week, or every two weeks, just to see where you are to help you stay on track. Or take photos to compare your front, side, and back every month and notice the positive changes in your physique. Notice how your clothes are fitting. That way, if you detect an unhealthy trend starting to develop, you can change up your regimen.

Cultivate Mindfulness

Mindfulness is a form of meditation that can help you relax both your mind and body and work through your anxiety, pain, and depression. Committing to mindfulness provides a comprehensive check-in for your mind and body to come together.

Being mindful can be as simple as stopping to take in a deep breath and notice what is happening around you. What are you feeling, seeing, hearing, smelling, touching, tasting? It's a form of "stopping to smell the roses" and can help you notice and enjoy the little things in life.

If you're feeling stressed, focus on the breath coming in and going out of your body. Close your eyes and be attentive to your deep breathing. If a thought comes into your mind, notice it and let it go, coming back to your breathing. The more you practice, the easier it becomes to tune in to yourself.

How Do I Find Support?

Keep in mind that finding a supportive community can look different for everyone. Here are some tips to help you stay supported.

Join a Fitness Support Group

Joining a fitness support group is a fantastic way to commune with others who share your goals. You'll be able to exchange encouragement, recipes, workouts, tips, tricks, and more.

When you engage with other people who have similar health and fitness goals, you'll find inspiration and advice that can make a real difference in your attitude and your progress. Helping others achieve their goals can also make you more resolute in your own goals as well.

To find them, check out your local community or fitness center, your neighborhood Facebook pages, community websites or the Resources (page 203) for more inspiration.

Try Something New

Maybe you've always wanted to go camping or kayaking, or there's a local mountaintop you've been eyeing for a while. Think creatively and become acquainted with exhilarating activities outside your usual workouts.

And, if you're not the social type, or you can't get out, try taking a class online. These classes can help you engage with your fitness goals and interact with other people. You'll feed off one another's energy while all doing the workout at the same time, fostering belonging and community.

Make it your mission to become acquainted with a new fitness activity. You'll feel empowered and recharged, and it will help broaden your fitness horizons.

Refresh Your Routine

While you're branching out, try exploring new activities with a fitness focus!

If you really enjoy biking, you may like taking a cross-country bicycling vacation. If you're interested in travel, you might enjoy walking tours of historic places. Maybe there is a famous mountain in another country that you'd like to tackle, or perhaps you'd enjoy swimming in an exotic lake.

Accountability Is a Strong Motivator

When you work out with others or sign up for a fitness challenge, you will have the desire to do your best and put your best foot forward. Not wanting to suffer embarrassment and not wanting to be the weak link in the group can make a difference in your level of effort (this is known as the Köhler effect).

And don't forget, a lot of those challenges have big prizes for the winners. That alone may be all the motivation you need!

Make Fitness a Friends-and-Family Affair

Working out with friends and family makes fitness fun. Whether it's the accountability of knowing they are depending on you to meet at a certain time, or the fact that you don't want to let another person down by not giving it your best effort, fitness, friends, and family go together. So, why not include your loved ones in your fitness lifestyle?

Try taking a nutritional cooking class with your partner or even become a coach for a child's or grandchild's sports team. Finding fitness-related activities that you both enjoy will help you spend quality time with each other as well as bond over common goals and activities.

How Do I Stay Motivated?

When you feel like giving up, having that list of "whys" you compiled at the beginning of this journey will help you stay on track and keep you motivated over the long term.

Remind yourself of the positive changes in your body, your energy levels, and your sleep quality, and build upon those successes.

Set an Appointment

Looking back, if you've found that it's been difficult to stick to your schedule, make adjustments. Consider choosing a different time to work out or perhaps another venue. Explore the things that have been getting in the way of regular exercise and get creative with ways to overcome these obstacles. Pick regular times of the week that will accommodate your workouts and coincide with your motivation and energy levels. Remember, if you set an appointment, it becomes a commitment.

Celebrate Your Progress

Keeping a journal to reflect upon your feelings can help you remember how you felt about yourself, physically and emotionally, throughout your fitness journey. Reflect on how you used to feel and compare that with how you feel and look now. Are you stronger? Do you have more endurance? Do you feel better, healthier, and more vibrant? Let yourself feel the boost in confidence that comes from the evidence of a job well done.

Also think about the lessons and the legacy you want to leave behind. Your offspring, friends, and family can all learn from you and your good example. Envision yourself being remembered as the picture of health, always able to show up for your family and friends. Being capable of participating in activities will leave a wonderful legacy.

Share Your Enthusiasm and Passion with Others

Perhaps you decided to hire a personal trainer to guide you at the beginning of this program and found that it helped you tremendously. Maybe it's time for you to pay it forward. Do you recall how nice it felt to be guided gently through your very first aerobics or yoga class? Do you want to help others feel that same level of comfort that you did?

Especially if you've fallen in love with a new fitness activity, consider getting certified as a trainer or instructor, or just showing others around your favorite gym, community center, or outdoor space. Why not continue the trend and share your success with others?

Set Another Goal

To pave the way for your success, make your goals SMART (specific, measurable, achievable, relevant, and timed) ones!

Be Specific. What is the ultimate outcome? Why is it important to you? Be detailed in describing it to yourself and to others!

Make It Measurable. For example, "I want to be able to do 10 push-ups by June 1." Measure your progress and accomplish mini goals along the way, but don't forget to set some big, long-term goals as well.

Make It Achievable. Make your goals challenging but not impossible. Set ambitious goals but be realistic.

Make It Relevant. Your goal should be meaningful to you, whether you want to hike the Appalachian Trail, run a marathon, or snowshoe in Alaska. Ensure it's important to you on multiple levels.

Make It Timed. Set mini deadlines and a final date for the full achievement of your goal. Use those progress points to check in throughout your journey and adjust course, if needed.

Reward Yourself

Once you have your goals in place, setting up rewards for yourself will also give you something to work toward. Have both smaller and larger non-food rewards for reaching mini deadlines and progress points, as well as more extensive rewards for getting to the finish line. You might start with something like a gold star on your calendar for every day that you stick to your plan. Choose things that will motivate you to stay on track.

This Is Just the Start

You now have the knowledge you need to take the next steps on your fitness journey. Best of all, you now know that you can do it! Keep up your momentum and keep moving forward in the direction you've chosen. Take it one day at a time and remember you're not trying to be perfect, just persistent. These healthy choices and changes will bring you a happier and healthier tomorrow. Congratulations on how far you've come, and welcome to the fitter you!

RESOURCES

Calculators and Scales

Free Dieting: FreeDieting.com

My Fitness Pal: MyFitnessPal.com

Ideal heart rate chart: Healthline.com/health/heart-disease
  /ideal-heart-rate#Ideal-heart-rate-for-exercise

Tips, Training Groups, and Tutorials

Tips for running a 5K race: The Couch 2 5K Running Program (C25k.com)

Find a Walking Group

VerywellFit.com/webwalking-usa-walking-program-3432830

AmericaWalks.org/tag/virtual-walks

Workout Tutorials

ACEFitness.org/education-and-resources/lifestyle/exercise-library

BodyBuilding.com/exercises

Fitness Books and Podcasts

Burn the Fat, Feed the Muscle by Tom Venuto

Jim Stoppani's Encyclopedia of Muscle & Strength by Jim Stoppani

Getting Stronger by Bill Pearl

A Guide to Flexible Dieting by Lyle McDonald

Found My Fitness by Rhonda Patrick, PhD: FoundMyFitness.com

Ben Greenfield Fitness: BenGreenfieldFitness.com/podcast

REFERENCES

Blumenthal, James A., Patrick J. Smith, Stephanie Mabe, Alan Hinderliter, Pao-Hwa Lin, Lawrence Liao, Kathleen A. Welsh-Bohmer, et al. "Lifestyle and neurocognition in older adults with cognitive impairments." *Neurology* 92, no. 3 (January 2019): e212–e223. n.Neurology.org/content/92/3/e212.

Erikson, Kirk I., Michelle W. Voss, Ruchika Shaurya Prakash, Chandramallika Basak, Amanda Szabo, Laura Chaddock, Jennifer S. Kim, et al. "Exercise training increases size of hippocampus and improves memory." *Proceedings of the National Academy of Sciences of the United States of America* 108, no. 7 (February 15, 2011): 3017–22.

Harvard Health Publishing. "The ideal stretching routine." Updated February 3, 2021. health.Harvard.edu/staying-healthy/the-ideal-stretching-routine.

Hrysomallis, Con. "Relationship between balance ability, training and sports injury risk." *Sports Medicine* 37, no. 6 (2007): 547–56. PubMed.NCBI.NLM.NIH.gov/17503879.

Krist, Lillian, Fernando Dimeo, and Thomas Keil. "Can progressive resistance training twice a week improve mobility, muscle strength, and quality of life in very elderly nursing-home residents with impaired mobility? A pilot study." *Clinical Interventions in Aging* 8 (April 23, 2013): 443–8. PubMed.NCBI.NLM.NIH.gov/23637524.

Marsman, D., D. W. Belsky, D. Gregori, M. A. Johnson, T. Low Dog, S. Meydani, S. Pigat, R. Sadana, A. Shao, J. C. Griffiths. "Healthy ageing: the natural consequences of good nutrition—a conference report." *European Journal of Nutrition* 57 (Suppl 2) (May 24, 2018): 15–34. PubMed.NCBI.NLM.NIH.gov/29799073.

Mortimer, James A., and Yaakov Stern. "Physical exercise and activity may be important in reducing dementia at any age." [Editorial] *Neurology* 92, no. 8 (February 19, 2019): 362–63. n.Neurology.org/content/92/8/362.

National Strength and Conditioning Association. "Benefits of flexibility training." *NSCA's Essentials of Personal Training, Second Edition*, Human Kinetics, May 2017. NSCA.com/education/articles/kinetic-select/benefits-of-flexibility-training.

Phillips, Stuart M., Stéphanie Chevalier, and Heather J. Leidy. "Protein 'requirements' beyond the RDA: implications for optimizing health." *Applied Physiology, Nutrition, and Metabolism* 41, no. 5 (May 2016): 565–72. PubMed.NCBI.NLM.NIH.gov/26960445.

Science Daily. "A lifetime of regular exercise slows down aging, study finds." Accessed February 20, 2021. ScienceDaily.com/releases/2018/03/180308143123.htm.

University of Rochester Medical Center. Calorie burn rate calculator. Accessed February 20, 2021. URMC.Rochester.edu/encyclopedia/content.aspx?ContentTypeID=41&ContentID=CalorieBurnCalc.

Wing, R. R., and R. W. Jeffery. "Benefits of recruiting participants with friends and increasing social support for weight loss and maintenance." *Journal of Consulting and Clinical Psychology* 67, no. 1 (February 1999): 132–38. PubMed.NCBI.NLM.NIH.gov/10028217.

INDEX

Acknowledgments

I thank God for the privilege of writing this book. Special thanks to my soul mate, Larry Waters, for supporting me in every way possible and helping me to clear my schedule to make this book happen.

Thank you to my family—Frank and Alrun Milligan; Antje and Tim Dew and Chloe, Sophie, and Micah Dew; Patsy Waters, John Waters, and Joe and Angela Waters—and for all my friends, both online and in person, who offered unwavering support and faith in me. And thank you to my coaches and mentors along the way. I have learned so much from you.

Thank you to my editor, Jesse Aylen, for being a pleasure to work with, and to Callisto Media for this fantastic opportunity.

About the Author

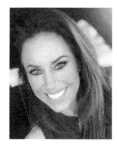

Stefanie Lisa was first introduced to weight lifting in college through a fitness book by Gladys Portugues called *Better Bodies*, and she became fascinated with the possibilities that weight lifting offered and how you could change the shape of your body and improve your physical health and mental outlook so vastly.

In 2009, she launched an online fitness and coaching company called Cougar Fitness with the aim of empowering people over 40 who have a desire to stay supple, fit, and healthy. The purpose of Cougar Fitness is to change the paradigms about age, as well as motivate, inspire, and teach others to be the best they can be at any age.

Fast-forward to many years after lifting that first dumbbell, and she has made fitness and healthy living her vocation. With her partner, Larry, and their fur babies, Skyelar and Thor, she enjoys a fitness lifestyle that includes bodybuilding, competing, and making the most of our "temples."

Her goal is to help you achieve your goals and live your best life, to be passionate about your health, and to live fit and be fierce.